Vivienne Parry is a scientist by training but an enthusiast by nature. She is best known as a presenter of BBC TV's popular science programme, *Tomorrow's World*, but for over fifteen years she was the National Organiser of the mother and baby research charity, WellBeing (formerly known as Birthright). She also writes for a wide variety of magazines and newspapers. She has two boys and lives with her house husband Paul in North London.

Her previous book, *The Antenatal Testing Handbook*, is also available in Pan.

By the same author

The Antenatal Testing Handbook

VIVIENNE PARRY

The Real Pregnancy Guide

in association with

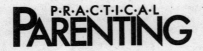

PAN BOOKS

This book is dedicated to the envelope-opening team: Nick, Jane, Oliver, Barney, Joshua and Clemency Keeler, Paul, Owen and Ellis Parry.

First published 1996 by Pan Books
an imprint of Macmillan General Books
25 Eccleston Place London SW1W 9NF
and Basingstoke

Associated companies throughout the world

ISBN 0 330 33285 6

1 3 5 7 9 8 6 4 2

A CIP catalogue record for this book is available from
the British Library.

Typeset by Parker Typesetting Service, Leicester
Printed by Mackays of Chatham plc, Chatham, Kent

Contents

Introduction

For over fifteen years, I was National Organiser of the mother and baby research charity WellBeing (formerly known as Birthright). I talked to thousands of women during my time there – on the phone, at meetings, in hospitals. I was struck by the number of conversations about pregnancy that began 'Why don't they tell you about . . .'. When I read pregnancy books, I began to understand what women meant. There was very little on 'real' pregnancy, as opposed to picture-book pregnancy, and almost nothing on pregnancy problems. I also began to realise that there were many things that worried women in pregnancy, which they felt unhappy discussing with their medical carers or even their friends – hence the number of calls that I, as an anonymous source of support, received over the years.

My experience was subjective, however, and I needed hard and fast data about what really worried women in pregnancy before I could set out to write the sort of book that would plug that gaping information gap. So with the splendid Helen Gill (then editor of *Practical Parenting* magazine), and with the financial support of Tesco plc, I set out to find what pregnancy was really about – from the horse's mouth, as it were – via a survey.

The survey 'What worries mums to be?' appeared in *Practical Parenting* in March 1994. We expected to have about 1,500 replies – we actually had not far short of 10,000, making it the most successful survey ever run in the magazine. The results of the survey appear in Appendix III.

But I was still reluctant. When I had written a previous book, on antenatal testing, it was reviewed in a magazine which was distributed to GPs. The doctor who wrote it was complimentary, but said that he thought that the majority of mothers would not welcome such detailed information. The inference was that 'not knowing' was preferable because 'knowing' would frighten women and cause unnecessary anxiety. I have always been aware that pregnant women are a uniquely vulnerable group, so with this, and the review, firmly in my mind, one of the questions included in the survey was 'Would you prefer not to know what could go wrong during pregnancy?'. Over 80 per cent of respondents, the overwhelming majority, said they would want to know.

Knowledge is enabling, not disabling. When we asked the question 'What did you wish you'd known before you got pregnant?', we were inundated with replies that said things like 'about caesarean sections', 'that births don't always go as you plan', 'about pre-eclampsia', 'about premature birth', 'about stitches'; indicating that there are many things that are not adequately explained to women. One shocking statistic emerged from the survey – that nearly half of our respondents felt, with hindsight, that they hadn't been properly prepared for what happened during labour.

It would have been easy, in writing a book in response to people's worries and concerns, to highlight the bad at the expense of the good. However, looking through all the thousands of survey replies, I am struck by women's honesty and good humour, and above all by the overwhelmingly positive messages about pregnancy that they wanted to give to other women. Yes, there are niggles, times when it isn't fun and even, for the unlucky few, dangers. But there are many real and splendid pleasures.

Some of these pleasures were physical – for instance, feeling the baby move was mentioned by almost every respondent. Even now, with my babies fast approaching adolescence, these comments about the baby moving very quickly took me back to pregnancy:

> 'The baby kicking – I sometimes used to stand there crying with happiness when it happened.'

> 'I couldn't take it all seriously until the baby started moving and then I just blossomed.'

> 'The kicking was wonderful, even though I did think he had boots on.'

> 'Those little bumps and flutters – glorious.'

> 'My husband holding me as the baby moved was one of the best things ever to have happened to me.'

Perhaps more surprisingly, many pleasures were psychological, with women finding that, particularly when pregnancy became very evident, they were the centre of attention. Here are just a few comments: 'I loved the way that strangers smiled at me'; 'it was the way that people treated me'; 'it was great telling everyone at work'; 'I enjoyed feeling special and the concern of my family and friends'; 'there was so much attention from so many people'. Whilst respect for the elderly and for the differences between men and women seem to have taken a battering over the last few years, it would appear that the sight of that bulge still seems to induce a universal respect and concern. And for all that we might argue, when not pregnant, that we want to be treated exactly the same as men, it takes pregnancy to convince us that being different and being cosseted and cared for can be a pretty special experience. For many of you the closeness that the growing life within you brings to the relationship with your partner was a particular joy.

We specifically asked about the relationship with your partner during pregnancy. About half of you said that the relationship was different in some way – with the overwhelming majority claiming that it was better. Was it because of hot sex – an increase in libido is reported by many pregnant women? Interestingly, only 16 per cent of you said that sex was better during pregnancy, which leads me to the inescapable conclusions that good loving isn't necessarily just about good sex, and that even if your sex life is less active, your relationship does not have to suffer. I make these points partly because, having read all those survey forms, I know just how many of you were concerned about the way in which lack of sex during pregnancy or after birth might affect the relationship with your partner. Take heart from this survey and know just how many women, despite their concern, discovered that their worries were unfounded. Stay close during pregnancy, experiment with different ways of loving that make you both feel special, and whatever you do, don't stop after delivery – you need each other more than ever.

Some of you evidently kept pregnancy to yourself, or to you and your partner, and very much enjoyed the pleasure that this secret gave you. Others blurted the whole thing out the minute the pregnancy test did its stuff – and whilst there were a few regrets because of this approach (mostly because of subsequent things that went wrong), by the time you reached the middle months of pregnancy you were all, whatever your early stance, pretty much thrusting your bump proudly before you, and loving it.

There were lots of other feelings that you enjoyed that you

wanted to tell other women about; 'the anticipation', 'all the planning and preparation' and 'feeling so very grown up' were some of the most common. And far from worrying all the time, some, like this woman, found that 'the time between the third month and the birth were the most relaxed and least worrying time of my life'. 'Looking back on it, the latter months of pregnancy had an almost dreamlike quality about them. Nothing phased me, I was on my own private cloud the whole time.'

One of the most wonderful things about pregnancy is the growing sense of your baby as a person. Sometimes this starts with the scan, sometimes it starts with the first kick. Some of the most special memories of pregnancy are of those very intimate moments when it's just you and your baby. 'I loved feeling her move when I sang to her in the bath'; 'I found I was talking to my baby out loud'; 'I patted my bump when I thought he needed reassuring'; and even this – 'I found myself asking him out loud whether he liked the colour of paint I was choosing for his bedroom'. Anyone who has never been pregnant may find this rather foolish, yet I know that anyone who has been pregnant or is pregnant now, will know exactly how magical such moments can be.

There are certainly times during pregnancy, particularly in the latter months, when your body does not look its best. Yet for all that, there were hundreds of comments on how good you looked and felt. For instance, because hair contains oestrogen receptors, it becomes glossier during pregnancy. In addition, very little hair falls out (it saves this up for after the birth) so it looks a lot thicker. Again because of high-circulating oestrogen levels, skin quality can improve dramatically, leading to comments like these: 'It was the first time in my life that my spots went'; 'I never had greasy hair'; 'my hair looked exactly like one of those adverts' and this, which I think was very sweet: 'my granddad said that my hair looked as pretty as it did when I was a little girl.'

As for weight – well, some of you get black marks for comments like these: 'I loved the rest of my overweight frame looking smaller'; 'I didn't have to pull my tummy in all the time'; 'I didn't worry about getting into my clothes once'; 'I never worried about my waistline once'. I'll lecture you at length later, but pregnancy is not a time to stuff yourself with any old rubbish on the 'it doesn't matter if I put on weight now' line. However, increasing weight, particularly around the bust, did bring a lot of pleasure to many. 'I had a bosom for the first time in my life'; 'I had a cleavage to die for'; 'Nell Gwynn had nothing on me, my partner went wild' – or 'If they'd got any bigger, I would have had to put lead in my shoes. It was great.' And having the opportunity (sorry, Freudian slip – necessity was the word you should be using to those around you) to go on a spree and buy new clothes was obviously hugely enjoyable. 'I bought new clothes and it really was a new me, like one of those makeovers.'

Finally, in terms of general health, many of you glowed for Britain. Not having periods was the most mentioned health benefit of pregnancy, with no PMT being a close second. An increased appetite and general level of fitness – 'I could have walked for miles' was a typical comment – were often mentioned. So too was the central heating effect of pregnancy: 'I loved being hot all the time when I'd always been frozen'; 'I was forever throwing off clothes instead of piling them on'; 'my feet were boiling instead of freezing'.

But the best things? Here are just a few:

'Seeing the baby on the scan for the first time.'

'Feeling the kicks.'

'Having the baby have hiccups inside me.'

'Buying the vests.'

As for advice from other mothers, it was interesting that over one-third of them said, in one way or another, 'Relax and enjoy it!' Here is a summary of all their advice – your ten-point plan to a happier pregnancy from nearly 10,000 other women:

1. Relax and enjoy it.
2. Get lots of rest and sleep and make the most of it while you can.
3. Try not to worry.
4. Follow your instincts and listen to your body.
5. Find out all you can and try to be informed.
6. Keep an open mind and expect anything.
7. Don't listen to other people's horror stories, all births are different.
8. Slow down, the housework can wait.
9. Never be afraid to ask questions.
10. Don't overeat – you'll regret it afterwards.

So don't be blinded by the number of pages on problems in this book and think that it must mean pregnancy is always difficult or alarming. Pregnancy is overwhelmingly a special time with moments of real joy for all women, and that's what came over, hurricane strength, from the readers of *Practical Parenting*. However, what also came across was the need for clear, non-patronising, sensible information about not just the little niggles, but the skated-over, you're-never-likely-to-have-them-so-don't-worry-about-them, big things. There is nothing worse than having your head stuck in the sand for you, only to be paralysed with fear for lack of information when you are finally obliged to come up for air. So this book is for you, from those readers of *Practical Parenting*, all of them mothers. All I have done is translate what they told me into a book for a new generation of mothers. I hope you find it helpful.

Vivienne Parry

1

Deciding to Have a Baby

You've seen it happen to your friends. You scoffed. Now it has happened to you. Perhaps it is the effect of time ticking on, perhaps it is the feeling of closeness and security that you and your partner have achieved together, perhaps it just feels right. Whatever the reason, the need (for such it is) to be pregnant and to have a baby has arrived. Somehow, something you had dismissed from your mind totally for so many years now becomes all consuming in a way that you had never imagined it would.

Whilst there are undoubtedly some women who plan pregnancy with all the thoroughness of a military campaign, getting 'fit' for pregnancy six months or so before conception, others are content just to smile that secret smile and sigh. You know immediately what is consuming their bedroom hours and that their 'planning' amounts simply to the knowledge that now is the time. Women who consciously think about getting pregnant are actually in the minority, with over 75 per cent of pregnancies worldwide being unplanned. You may find that statistic shocking, especially if you are one of those who planned, or are planning their pregnancies (and if you are reading this book, it is a pretty fair guess that you are one of these – almost all our *Practical Parenting* survey respondents had planned their pregnancies). You may feel that you have the moral high ground – how could women not think ahead about something so important? In truth, whilst planning is important, real life has a way of dispensing with the best laid plans, of bowling a googly at the most unexpected moments and of making a mockery of your aspirations and hopes – which is how many of us get pregnant in the first place. Time, chance, passion and our reproductive cycles conspired – and caught up with each other.

Planning ahead does not guarantee that things will go well, as we all know from experience. It may reduce risks but it cannot eliminate risk altogether, much in the same way that checking the oil level in the car before you go on a long journey might prevent your engine seizing up, but doesn't stop a runaway lorry totalling your car just around the next corner. This is not to diminish the benefits of planning for a pregnancy but an attempt to put it into context. If you are already pregnant, you may read the remainder of this chapter with growing dismay, fearing that because you were unable to plan, for whatever reason, something is bound to go wrong. Again, you have to put things in context. To go back to the car analogy, how often have you failed to check your oil level, but still managed to reach your destination safely?

Pregnancy outcome is very rarely decided on a single swing of the pendulum. Instead, it is rather like a game with one of those old-fashioned balances, built on the Scales of Justice model. Around this balance are hundreds of different weights, some small, some large, some overwhelming in size, representing the different factors affecting the success or otherwise of an individual pregnancy. For some women, who have many positives on their balance, a few negatives may make little difference. Of course smoking is harmful, but it has less of an effect in a mother who is well nourished than in a poorly nourished woman who has a high alcohol and caffeine intake. On the other hand, you can have all the positives in the world on one side and still have them outweighed by the unknown negatives contained in your or your baby's genes.

Planning ahead may not be a guarantee of a healthy baby, but there is one thing that it can guarantee – peace of mind. If you are consciously planning pregnancy, you suddenly become much more aware of potential hazards. You don't take medicines without grilling your doctor first as to their advisability in pregnancy; you eat well, think about your health, and drink orange juice on hen nights instead of going for broke with the Babycham. In this way you avoid the trauma faced by those women who, not knowing they were pregnant, inadvertently took medicines, neglected their diets and health and generally Had a Good Time. On discovering they are pregnant, these women are completely traumatised by guilt and worry for the rest of their pregnancy.

Or even after the birth, in the case of one woman I met who had had no idea she was pregnant, despite having had two children before. She was admitted to hospital with acute abdominal pain and examined by a coterie of puzzled doctors on the gynaecological ward who diagnosed a ruptured ovarian cyst, only for an alert medical student to whisper to the consultant, 'I don't like to alarm you, sir, but there's a head between her legs.' Truly. I very much doubt that any of the distraught women I spoke to over the years at WellBeing who had unplanned pregnancies had babies that were anything but normal; nevertheless, their pregnancies were ruined by anxiety. Advance planning prevents this.

Much of the advice, then, that follows comes into the category of 'I wish I'd known'. So much of it was echoed by our survey respondents with pre-conception diet (in particular the need for folic acid supplements) and being fit before getting pregnant being paramount. One thing that you can't do (although a worrying number of people think they can) is say when you are going to get pregnant; it might be immediate, it might take six months, it might take a year. Whatever you do in preparation has to be a lifestyle change, not a blitzkrieg course in monastic abstention, because for sure and certain you won't be able to keep that up for six months.

So, reconsider your lifestyle, not only because you want to have a baby but because soon, if things work out as you hope, you will have a family. Your health practices will soon be theirs, not just for their childhood but for the rest of their lives. Remember, however, that the suggestions here as to what you do prior to, and during, pregnancy represent an optimum lifestyle, not the only lifestyle to result in successful pregnancy.

Physical Fitness

'I wish I'd been fitter, I'm sure I would have coped better.'

'I wish I'd known how much pregnancy takes it out of you.'

'I never bothered about exercise before my first pregnancy but I vowed I'd be fit for the second. What a difference!'

Some time ago, an eminent obstetrician compiled a pre-pregnancy guide called *Getting Fit to be Pregnant*. It suggested that you should run at least a mile a day. Dutifully, my friend and I advanced into the park at lunchtime. She held the stopwatch and I did the running. She got pregnant and I put my back out.

Actually, being able to run a mile in four minutes dead isn't what it's all about. In fact, just the opposite. Very heavy exercise will result in a large proportion of body fat being replaced with muscle tissue. Under these circumstances, ovulation is affected and periods may become irregular. Up to a quarter of female cross-country and marathon runners, and four out of five ballet dancers, have irregular periods because of this. Generally, periods (and ovulation) return to normal with a small reduction in the amount of exercise and a small increase in body weight (of about 5 per cent). If after six months or so they are not back to normal, medical help should be sought.

There are several other situations related to body weight, in which ovulation will be affected. If you are too thin you will not ovulate normally because ovulation mechanisms depend, as I have just outlined, on having a critical mass of body fat. Being overweight will also affect your cycles. In women who have polycystic ovaries (a cause of irregular periods and also fertility problems) it has been shown that losing weight (very often these women are overweight) will not only restore their periods to something approaching normal but also improve fertility. Fiddling about with those height-for-weight charts can be a bit of a trial, since they vary enormously and are open to all that 'but I'm big boned' nonsense we all resort to when faced with such things. A better measure is your body mass index (BMI), which you calculate by dividing your weight in kilograms by the square of your height in metres – you should come out with a figure between 20 and 25. Over, and you need to lose weight; under, and you need to gain some. Nor should you neglect your partner in all this ideal weight business, because there have been several studies which show a decline in sperm quality with obesity.

Being fit for pregnancy has two main aims. The first is to do with the health of your baby and the second is all about you. Let's deal with you first. Pregnancy is hugely demanding. If you are puffing after running up the stairs now, think what it

Are you the correct weight for your height?

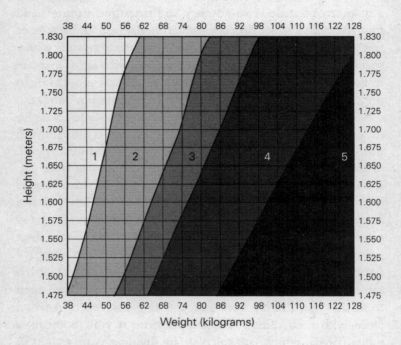

Band 1 = underweight
Band 2 = normal weight
Band 3 = overweight
Band 4 = fat
Band 5 = very fat

Are you the correct weight for your height?

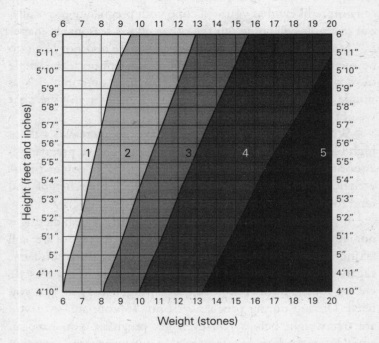

will be like when you are carrying another couple of stone. Being in good shape, with good muscle tone, with the sort of energy levels that regular exercise brings with it, makes it not only more likely that you will cope with pregnancy physically, but that you will come out the other side in reasonable shape.

Now to the baby. If you are fit, you are also not likely to be overweight. A mother's weight at conception is the single most important determining factor in fetal outcome. It's as simple as that. Not overweight, not underweight, just the right weight for your height.

Women who are overweight have an increased risk of high blood pressure, of premature delivery, and of pregnancy-associated diabetes. Their babies tend to be of lower birth-weight. Women who are underweight for their height also tend to have lighter babies.

If you are overweight, think about dieting. Crash dieting is not appropriate. You need to make sure that you are still taking all the necessary nutrients whilst cutting down on fatty, sugary food and taking more exercise. As I said, it is a lifestyle change for the future not just a quick weight-loss plan that you need. Dieting during pregnancy is not appropriate, so if you are overweight before you even get pregnant, you have an awful lot of work to do afterwards. In our survey more women were worried about putting on weight they wouldn't lose than they worried about going into premature labour. When we asked 'What did you enjoy about pregnancy?', quite a few people said 'not having to hold my stomach in' and 'not having to diet'. Try losing it before, and don't be despondent if it takes a bit of time. Of course you are also more likely to conceive quickly if you are an ideal weight. If you are underweight, you will need to think about gaining a few pounds.

A final caveat on being overweight and blood pressure.

Women with high blood pressure may also retain fluid to an alarming degree (oedema). Water weighs heavy, and in these cases the weight gain is a consequence of high blood pressure, not a cause of it.

SMOKING

Women often ask me about the best type of diet prior to and during pregnancy, and about what type of vitamin supplements they should be taking. In the course of the conversation, I discover that they are heavy smokers. Never mind the vitamin pills; giving up smoking is infinitely more important in terms of the health of your baby, both during pregnancy and for the future. Smoking is a well-documented cause of infertility, miscarriage and premature labour. Babies born to smokers are smaller, and at greater risk of death. Your unborn baby is directly affected by your smoking. Cot death, asthma, breathing problems and hearing difficulties (caused by glue ear) are all more common in babies who live in households where someone smokes.

Get a grip on yourself now. Don't just resolve to cut down prior to pregnancy. Give it up. Having had a totally addicted, fifty-a-day mother, I know, however, that giving it up is pretty hard. If you need help, phone Quitline, the telephone helpline for QUIT – see Appendix I. There are several good paperbacks on how to stop available from bookshops, and lots of treatment aids such as nicotine chewing gum. Incidentally, this latter is contra-indicated in pregnancy, so giving up smoking is a project that is best taken on whilst you are still using contraceptives.

Nor should this be a project which you approach on your own. Heavy smoking is known to affect sperm quality in men, and having their father smoke is just as unhealthy for your newborn baby as having their mother smoke, so get your partner involved, give each other moral support, and aim to make this a lifestyle change for you as well as a health measure for your baby.

ALCOHOL

The Health Education Authority now recommends an upper limit of 21 units of alcohol a week for women. All available evidence is that there should be an upper limit of 8 units of alcohol per week for pregnant women with no more than 2 units being consumed in any one day (a unit is half a pint of ordinary strength beer or lager, a glass of red or white wine or a pub measure of spirits), but the less you drink during pregnancy the better. Alcohol is a poison which crosses the placenta and directly affects the baby. Some, but not all, babies born to alcoholic mothers are affected by Fetal Alcohol Syndrome, in which there is a characteristic range of physical malformations as well as learning difficulties.

Whilst women planning pregnancy may cut down their alcohol intake, it is true to say that a great many babies (who knows, perhaps the majority) are conceived in a slightly alcoholic haze. Women who got pregnant in this way often think that their babies may be affected. It is possible to be very reassuring, however. For the first two weeks of its existence, before implantation is completed, the fertilised egg is incredibly resistant to insult. If the insult is great enough to cause damage, implantation does not occur and that's that – no pregnancy. The very fact that your pregnancy continued implies that all was well. Binge drinking during periods of organ formation sensitive to alcohol may be another story, but unfortunately determining how much drink constitutes dangerous binge drinking, or what are the sensitive periods, is very difficult; there are so many ifs and buts and, frankly, so many conflicting studies. Probably the most sensible thing is to say that an occasional drink is unlikely to harm your baby, but that you would be best keeping alcohol intake to a minimum.

I once received a long letter from a lady concerned about some minor problem of pregnancy. The crux of the letter, however, was the PS at the bottom: 'Will my baby be an alcoholic because my husband was drunk when the baby was conceived?' I wrote to the woman saying that her husband couldn't have been that drunk, and that she was not to worry.

However, there are concerns for men too. Heavy drinking is known to affect performance – but it can also affect sperm counts. A study at the Royal Free Hospital in London (which admittedly only involved small numbers) showed an increased sperm count when previously heavy drinkers laid off the booze. The mechanisms of how alcohol might affect sperm quality are various and include a disruption of the hormonal pathways between the testes and the hypothalamus (the hormonal master conductor), a mutagenic effect on sperm, and even, for beer drinkers, an oestrogenic or feminising effect caused by the hops in beer which are apparently quite strongly oestrogenic. And of course, drinking involves lots of calories and usually a fair amount of excess weight which is, as I have outlined, known in itself to affect sperm quality.

FOLATE

Apart from the sort of lifestyle diet changes I have spoken about, which do just as much for you as they do for your baby, there are some specific dietary considerations, prior to pregnancy.

'I wish I'd known about folate.'

'Why isn't everybody told about folic acid supplements now?'

Folate, a B group vitamin which is also called folic acid, is present in a wide variety of foods. The richest sources are green leafy vegetables such as spinach, broccoli and Brussels sprouts (fresh or frozen). It is also found in potatoes, oranges and Marmite. Many types of bread and cereal also contain quite large quantities if they have been fortified (you know which ones these are because they list the vitamin levels on the side of the packet; the unfortified ones probably have more vitamins in the cardboard box than in the cereal itself). A bowl of fortified breakfast cereal contains a quarter of the recommended daily intake of folate.

For many years there has been a running controversy as to whether supplements of folic acid prevent neural tube defects (NTDs – the family of handicaps which includes spina bifida and anencephaly). It has been shown that in women who have had a previous baby with an NTD, the subsequent incidence is reduced by about 70 per cent if folate supplements are given. It has now been suggested that all women should take folic acid supplements around the time of conception. Just because a lot is good for some does not necessarily mean that a little is good for everyone, although this appears to be what the Department of Health is saying. Neural tube defects are known to be multi-factorial in origin – in other words, no one thing causes them but a mixture of factors, some inherited and some environmental (which would explain the wide variation in prevalence in Britain). It is possible that women who have babies with NTDs are unable to metabolise folate as effectively as other women, but until it is feasible to identify them in advance it makes sense to suggest supplementation to everyone, although, as I have suggested, it is a bit of a leap in thinking.

All women who are planning a pregnancy are now advised to take a daily supplement of 400 mcg of folic acid prior to conception, and during the first three months. In addition it is suggested that they have a folate rich diet. At first, 400 mcg supplements were not available on prescription, despite it being the Department of Health which was recommending taking them. They are now, but since the prescription is not free (because you are not yet pregnant) the prescription charge actually costs more than the tablets, which you would be better off buying direct from health food shops or your local chemist. Women who have had a previous baby affected by an NTD are advised to take a much higher dosage of folate, 5 mg daily, and this is only available on prescription. Similar advice applies to those with an NTD in the family.

You might be tempted to take much larger doses than recommended. Don't be. It is known that increasing the intake of some minerals affects the uptake of others (for instance, extra zinc intake causes a fall in iron uptake by the body). Nobody is yet sure what effect large amounts of folate have on the body, although there seems to be no evidence of harm at present, so be cautious. You can of course try to take in the maximum recommended daily intake of folate of 700 mcg (i.e. 300 mcg from food and 400 mcg supplement) all from food, but it is surprisingly hard to do, at least on a consistent basis, without shifting broccoli faster than a Covent Garden porter. You may be a confirmed broccoli hater and, if already pregnant, feeling deeply alarmed because your folate intake wasn't up to much in the early months of pregnancy. Please don't worry. The incidence of spina bifida has been falling for some years and these handicaps remain rare. In addition, routine screening is offered during pregnancy. Finally, the fact that folic acid supplementation does not totally prevent births of babies with NTDs should tell you that lack of folate is just part of the NTD picture, not the whole story.

IRON

Because of the increase in blood volume during pregnancy, large quantities of iron are required to form the oxygen-carrying blood pigment, haemoglobin, and good stores of iron are essential to healthy pregnancy. Most women should have reasonable iron stores prior to pregnancy. However, those with very heavy periods may have low iron stores, as may vegetarians and vegans, since iron is more readily absorbed from meat than from other foods. Worryingly, some recent surveys have revealed that many women have a lower daily intake of iron than that recommended. You may need to think about iron supplements prior to pregnancy, therefore, if you are a vegetarian or if you have particularly heavy periods.

Iron supplementation during pregnancy is a vexed question. Originally, supplements were given routinely because the level of iron in the blood fell quite dramatically during pregnancy. However, this is largely because the blood increases in volume, thus diluting the amount of iron, rather than because there is a deficiency. Iron is unpleasant to take, causing nausea, indigestion and constipation in many women, and there is much evidence to suggest that most iron supplements end up down the pan. Thus, supplements are now reserved for those women who show evidence of iron deficiency. Prior to pregnancy, you might like to think of ways to increase the amount of iron that you take in, by some simple alterations to your eating habits. Drinks containing vitamin C increase the amount of iron absorbed from iron-containing foods, whilst tea and coffee reduce it. Iron absorption is also reduced by eating wholegrains and soya products. This is an important consideration for vegetarians, who may already have an iron-restricted diet. Many soya products are now iron fortified, and if you are a vegetarian it might be preferable to use these.

SUPPLEMENTING WITH OTHER VITAMINS AND MINERALS

One recent study in Hungary has shown a decrease in malformations at birth in babies born to women who had supplements of multivitamins around conception. You may think that you might as well take a vitamin supplement, just to be on the safe side; and this is a reasonable assumption. Nevertheless, it is far better to get your vitamins from your food and from a balanced diet than to get them out of a bottle, especially if taking supplements means that you neglect proper consideration of your diet. Also, vitamin intake isn't just a question of swallowing the right pills; absorption is regulated by complex interactions between different foods eaten in the diet – like the vitamin C and iron story above. Finally, be aware of the dosage of additional vitamins you are taking as it is quite easy to overdose, especially on the fat-soluble vitamins A and D.

Vitamin A is particularly suspect. It comes in two forms: retinol (from animal sources) and carotene (from plant sources). High doses of carotene are not harmful, whilst high intakes of retinol are very toxic. Arctic explorers who ate the livers of polar bears (which contain large amounts of retinol) to survive, died, fatally poisoned by vitamin A. A number of birth defects have been linked with excessive vitamin A intake in the first three months of pregnancy. The recommendation from the Department of Health is that pregnant women should be consuming not more than 3,300 mcg (11,000 IU) of retinol daily. This means that you should avoid taking fish oil supplements (except those manufactured from the body of the fish, rather than from the liver) and also avoid eating liver, or liver products such as pâté, because of their high retinol content. Remember too that many everyday foods such as bread and cereals are fortified with vitamins, adding quite considerably to your daily intake.

I am often asked about this by women who have inadvertently eaten liver before they knew they were pregnant. It is possible to be very reassuring; yet these women often say, with good reason, that if reassurance is possible, why are they told not to eat it? The answer is that in making recommendations there is always a tendency to err well on the side of caution, leaving a wide margin of safety.

SPECIAL DIETS

Traditional Asian diets are often low in calcium and contain many wholewheat foods, such as chapatis, which are high in phytate which inhibits calcium absorption. Calcium supplements prior to and during pregnancy may therefore be appropriate. Asian diets may also contain inadequate amounts of vitamin D. Because many Muslim women cover their heads and bodies, the alternative source of vitamin D, via the skin through the action of sunlight, is not available to them either. Asian women are recommended to take a 10 mcg supplement daily of vitamin D.

Vegetarian diets may be low in B12, which is only obtained from animal sources. Strict vegetarians may require additional magnesium, since compounds in vegetable proteins can bind the mineral, thus making it useless. Vegans may have special problems in fulfilling their needs for calcium, magnesium and vitamin D as well as for B12. If you are macrobiotic, you may have to rethink your diet completely, as the macrobiotic regime does not provide enough calcium or protein, lacks the necessary nutrients found in fruit and is inappropriate for pregnancy. Adding fish, tofu and fruit to the diet, as well as a calcium supplement, is a first step.

It is as well to think of these things before you get pregnant, not only because the last thing that you want to be doing when you may be feeling sick and miserable in the first few weeks of pregnancy is radically adjusting your diet, but also because you are building up stores of nutrients which will sustain you and the baby in those first few vital months.

Other Considerations

CONTRACEPTION

Some books solemnly advise women to give up the pill in favour of barrier methods of contraception at least six months prior to conception. Several reasons are advanced. The first is that the pill affects fertility and time is needed to restore full fertility; the second is that time is required to 'clear the system' of hormones, or the baby will be adversely affected; third is that the pill affects nutritional status. I think mythconceptions is probably the term to apply to all of these statements.

> 'I was expecting it to take at least six months to conceive. I wish I'd known it was going to be a "hole in one", the first time we made love after I came off the pill!'

Women seem to be more aware of those who have come off the pill and subsequently had fertility problems than women who come off the pill and get pregnant immediately, even though the latter is much more common. The pill is a reversible method of birth control. Whilst there are some women who have problems with periods, or even no periods, when they stop the pill, these are no more common than in comparable women who do not take the pill. It is probably the case that these women would have suffered from menstrual disturbances, but that the regular withdrawal bleeds provided by the pill masked their condition. It is the case, however, that women in their thirties take longer to conceive if they have been on the pill than women who have used barrier methods of birth control, although conception rates eventually become identical in the two groups. Fertility is not affected by length of use of the pill, nor is it ameliorated by 'breaks' from the pill. Many women find that they are particularly fertile in the few months after stopping the pill.

Some women manage to get pregnant even though they are on the pill. They naturally worry that the pill will harm their baby. No woman can be promised a healthy baby, since at least 2 per cent of babies will have a serious abnormality. The Population Council estimated that 7 *out of every 10,000 pregnancies exposed to the pill might have a possibly attributable abnormality*. To put this in perspective, this would increase the background rate by 0.1 per cent, i.e. from 2 per cent to 2.1 per cent. In 1990, a summary of all available data concluded that exposure to oral contraceptives did not increase the risk of anomalies over that in non-exposed populations. But is there any residual risk to the baby for pill users? The balance of published work is heavily tilted towards complete absence of risk. My friend with the unexpected baby had taken the pill throughout her pregnancy – her baby was just fine.

Finally there is some concern that the pill alters vitamin levels, especially B vitamins and vitamin C, and also reduces zinc levels, and that this in itself might be a potential cause of harm to the baby. This was more notable when women were using the older, high dosage pills, than it is today. There is no evidence that these alterations in blood levels are likely to cause any problems, and in any case values quickly return to normal once the pill is discontinued. If you want to be pessimistic about the pill, give it up a couple of months in advance, but more is not necessary. It used to be said that another reason for doing this was to establish your periods and thus be sure of being able to date your pregnancy accuracy (pregnancies are dated from the first day of the last period). However, as ultrasound can now do this very well, this is no longer a concern.

RUBELLA STATUS

All pregnant women are tested at their booking-in visit to hospital to see whether they are immune to rubella (German measles). A surprising number turn out not to be immune, despite having had a rubella vaccination as a teenager. Rubella is a very common virus in the community and, particularly if you either work with children or have other children, you are quite likely to come across it during pregnancy. For heaven's sake, save yourself the agony and double-check your rubella immunity before you get pregnant.

TOXOPLASMA

You might also consider having testing for toxoplasma status prior to pregnancy. *Toxoplasma gondii* is a parasite whose main host is the domestic cat. Humans can become infected with toxoplasma causing an illness called toxoplasmosis, which is usually trivial. But if women become infected during pregnancy, there is a risk that the infection will pass to the baby. Although there is more chance of the infection being passed to the baby later in pregnancy, there is more chance of the baby being affected in early pregnancy. About 10 per cent of infected babies have severe problems, typically hydrocephalus (fluid on the brain), scarring of brain tissue (which may result in brain damage) and blindness. A proportion of infected babies who are perfectly normal at birth go on to develop a specific type of eye problem, which may result in blindness in later life. This sounds very alarming, but you have to put it in perspective. The numbers of babies affected are small, perhaps even smaller than experts might suggest. About 2 in every 1,000 women will catch toxoplasma in pregnancy. If this is right, it should result in 500–600 cases of congenital infection each year, of which about 60 cases would be severe. In fact the British Paediatric Surveillance Unit found a much smaller number of severely affected babies (about 10 in England and Wales per year). Are lots of affected babies being missed, or are they not being followed up for long enough, or is toxoplasma not such an extensive problem as was previously thought? No matter what numbers are involved, many women are sufficiently concerned to have asked for toxoplasma testing in pregnancy. The results are often confusing, with large numbers of false positives. In addition, the blood tests don't tell you what you want to know, which is 'has my baby been affected?', rather than 'has my baby been infected?'. Say you are six months pregnant and the tests show evidence of a past infection – was it contracted three months before you got pregnant (stop panicking) or a month afterwards?

Knowing your toxoplasma antibody status prior to pregnancy can be sanity saving. Although as I have indicated there is a problem with false positives, both positive and negative toxoplasma antibody results prior to pregnancy should be treated in the same way. You should note the result and then follow all the simple hygiene rules (which actually are straight common sense anyway) in order to minimise any danger of infection during pregnancy.

Toxoplasma cysts do not become infective until forty-eight hours after being passed by an infected cat. Once the cat has been infected, it is immune thereafter. Since cats mostly catch this infection from mice and birds, most are immune by the time they reach adulthood (if they have been allowed to roam outside that is). Having an elderly moggy is not a reason to be concerned about toxoplasma. You should be careful with kittens, and cats that are not known to you. However, you actually have to swallow the infective toxoplasma cysts in order to become infected yourself, and providing you wash your hands after handling cats there is no reason why you should become infected – in any case, infective cysts are not usually found on the fur.

This is a classic example of a piece of advice which, whilst well-intentioned, has got out of hand. Women frequently ask whether they should get rid of their cats because they are pregnant; I hope you now realise that the answer is a resounding no. Also, the advice not to touch cats has been interpreted to mean that toxoplasma can somehow be absorbed by skin contact with a cat. It can't.

Much of this advice, and I am now about to get on a favourite hobby horse of mine, is to do with basic hygiene – the sort of things that we should be doing anyway, not just in order to avoid toxoplasmosis or food poisoning. Dispose of cat litter regularly, wearing gloves. Wash your hands afterwards. Wear gloves when gardening and wash your hands before eating (told you it was basic) and wash soil from vegetables and salads before eating. In addition, because infective cysts can be transmitted via undercooked meat, you should make sure that you keep meat preparation areas separate from other cooking, wash your hands thoroughly after preparation and cook your meal thoroughly right through. If you must eat raw or undercooked meat, use meat that has previously been deep frozen to at least $-20°C$. Finally, because goat's milk sometimes contains toxoplasma, you should not drink it unless it has been pasteurised.

Many of the measures above, as I said, are common sense. Adapting your lifestyle should mean that you think about all aspects of your health, adopting practices which may be simple, such as washing your hands before and after food preparation, but which will stand you and your family in good stead for the rest of your lives.

DRUGS AND MEDICINES

Ever since the thalidomide tragedy, there is one message that women have received loud and clear: 'It is dangerous to take medicines in pregnancy.' There is no doubting the importance of this, but it has perhaps been overzealously interpreted, with many women now believing that almost any drug taken around the time of conception and in the early months of pregnancy will cause malformation. In truth there are only a handful of drugs that are proven teratogens (substances capable of causing fetal malformation). Also, in just the same way that one woman has side-effects if she takes the pill, whilst her friend has none, no two babies necessarily react in the same way to a particular teratogen. To exert its teratogenic effect (if it has one), a medicine has to be taken at the precise time in the baby's development when organs which are sensitive to the teratogen are being formed. For example, whilst a medicine might cause hearing problems in the baby if taken on day 25 of pregnancy, it might have no effect if taken on day 24 or day 26. Before 14 days, there is an all-or-nothing response to insult, as I have indicated.

The *British National Formulary* (BNF) is published every six months by the British Medical Association and the Royal Pharmaceutical Society, and is available in the reference section of your local library or through the BMA. It lists all licensed drugs and has an appendix which gives all those drugs which may have harmful effects on pregnancy. Many new drugs are automatically listed as not being suitable for use in pregnancy. This does not necessarily mean that they are dangerous, it just means that they haven't been tested for use in pregnancy, which isn't the same thing at all.

Knowing that you have taken medicines inadvertently is very worrying, but it is not uncommon for women to be taking antibiotics (particularly for urinary tract infections), the pill and a range of other medications when they get pregnant. The vast majority of these women will have normal babies. Of course it is better not to take medicines if you can help it, and here again you can see why planning ahead can save you infinite worry.

HAVING ANOTHER BABY TOO QUICKLY

Birth interval – the time between one baby and the next – is another considerable influence on fetal outcome, although this is less important in Western society where women are better nourished and where breast feeding tends to be of shorter duration. If you have decided that you want another baby very quickly (less than a year later), or if this is the way that it worked out, there is an increased risk of the next being born prematurely and/or of having low birthweight. You will need to pay special attention to your diet, and vitamin supplements may be important.

EXISTING MEDICAL CONDITIONS

Pre-planning is essential if you have a medical condition such as epilepsy, severe asthma, diabetes, heart or renal conditions, or if you are taking long-term medication, e.g. for high blood pressure. Whereas in the past pregnancy was sometimes not advised, modern care means that women can still have babies despite their medical conditions. However, two things are required – forethought and teamwork. First the teamwork. Your specialist consultant, be it a cardiologist or a neurologist, needs to work with you and with an obstetrician (preferably in the same hospital) to ensure that your condition is stable prior to pregnancy and that you get the best possible specialist advice and care during pregnancy and labour. Forethought means thinking about your drug regime (alternative drugs might be more appropriate in pregnancy); it means asking all the questions you want so that you appreciate all the implications of pregnancy; and it means a greater emphasis on your health and those special aspects of care to which you need to devote greater attention.

PROBLEMS IN PREVIOUS PREGNANCIES

You may feel particularly concerned about pre-conceptual care if you have had a previous pregnancy end in the loss of your baby. There may, in fact, be very little in medical terms that you can do to prevent whatever it was happening again, and you may find this lack of control particularly distressing. You may feel that if only you had done things differently before your previous pregnancy, your loss wouldn't have occurred. Often there is no rational basis for this kind of thinking (see Chapter 8 on miscarriage), but the need to do something positive for the next pregnancy is nevertheless of paramount importance in helping you cope. You may decide to do as much as you possibly can in the pre-conception period, treating it rather like an insurance policy. If it makes you feel good about the next time, then it has achieved its purpose and it has been well worthwhile – but don't see it as a copper-bottomed guarantee which will prevent loss occurring again.

The type of loss you suffered may decide your future medical care – for instance you may need high tech intervention from an early stage of pregnancy. You may feel very happy to continue with the same medical carers as before. On the other hand you may feel, particularly if communication was a problem, that you need a change. If this is the case, talk it over with your GP, ask him or her to refer you to a different consultant if necessary, or even to another hospital. Take the time to talk about your fears and worries, particularly with your partner, who may be more scared than you are but desperately trying to keep a lid on his concerns. You should both talk to the person who will be looking after you, be it GP or consultant, and discuss all the options. Write down all your concerns before you meet and try to go through all of them. The best doctors will be happy to go through all the options, and in particular will be clear about the risks of the same thing happening again, rather than just woolly reassurers.

There isn't a right time to think about getting pregnant again, but you both need to be ready before you try. With a late pregnancy loss you need to give your body more time to recover physically than with an earlier pregnancy loss. Early or late, you need time to come to terms with your loss. Only you will know when you are ready to try again.

Finally, there are a number of organisations which offer pre-conceptual care of one sort or another, claiming that if you take their very expensive pills and potions you will be guaranteed a healthy baby. No one can guarantee anything of the sort. And when they say things like 'our mothers don't have miscarriages with our supplements' (as I have heard), just remember that after one miscarriage, nine out of ten women will have a healthy baby next time round – no pills, no potions, no magic; that's just the way it is.

2

How to Get Pregnant

'I wish I'd known that you can be on the pill for seventeen years and get pregnant within a month. I spent at least ten years secretly worrying that it wouldn't happen.'

'Why does no one ever tell you that it takes a long time to get pregnant?'

'It was a hole in one. I went hot and cold thinking of all the times we'd been a bit negligent about contraception as students. How had we got away with it?'

'I was so disappointed that it didn't happen straightaway. I thought there was something wrong with me.'

'It took us over a year and by the end of it, I think my husband would have been happy if we'd never made love again. He hated me making him make love to order and it caused all sorts of stress and arguments.'

'I dreaded getting my period and knowing that yet again, I wasn't pregnant. It took about four months, but it seemed like forever. I never would have coped if it had taken longer.'

You would think, wouldn't you, that by the time you are big and grown up, you'd know how to get pregnant. A surprising number of people don't. Part of the problem, I think, is that there are two versions of the reproduction process. One of these was dinned into us at school. It ran something along the lines of: 'Make love at any time of your cycle, even during your period, and you could get pregnant.' It scared the knickers off us, as I recall, and we genuinely believed that if a penis (let along an erect one) came closer than about three feet, pregnancy would be instantaneous. By the time we get to the age of thirty or so, however, the advice has completely changed: 'You'll only get pregnant if you make love in your fertile period.' It is very difficult for most people to reconcile these two views in their minds and it leads to a great deal of disappointment and unhappiness.

Part of the difference, of course, is age – you are simply red hot in your youth, conception-wise that is. Fertility starts to decline most steeply after the age of about 30–31, with women of 40 being only about 25 per cent as fertile as women of 20. There are a number of reasons for this decline; one of the most obvious is that the older you get, the less likely you are to make love often. Robert Winston has produced a fascinating table to back this fact in his book *Getting Pregnant* (Pan, 1993). It shows that in Australia women make love on average 17.2 times a month when aged between 16–20, whereas frequency of lovemaking falls to just 6.8 times a month at the age of 40. In Britain it appears we are less sexually active when young: 9.9 times a month between 16–20, but by 35–39 we too are only making love half as often. If you are in your late thirties and reading this, you may console yourself with the fact that women reach their sexual peak at 40, and that the rate of multiple orgasm increases with age. So it may not be as often, but when it happens it's great. Other reasons for declining fertility with age are that ovulation may not occur as often, and that even if conception does occur, the embryo may not implant because eggs are of increasingly poor quality as women get older.

So how long should it take to get pregnant? The average British couple takes about six months, but it is perfectly normal for a quarter of British couples to take a year to conceive. About 10 per cent of couples will not conceive within a two-year period. Six months may seem like a lifetime to you, and you may become increasingly frustrated and disappointed when pregnancy does not occur.

You may have decided that you want to get pregnant quickly and that you should therefore only make love during your fertile period, in order to give yourselves the best possible chance of conception. So you may have got out the thermometer and be taking your temperature every day in an effort to detect when you are ovulating. You might also have bought one of those kits that has a urine dipstick which will tell you when you are about to ovulate. Furthermore, you may have been told that if you make love too often, your partner will 'exhaust' his sperm, or that he needs a period of abstinence from lovemaking in order to have top quality sperm for conception. So you may be holding your partner off with a barge-pole for much of your cycle, but locking him in the broom cupboard, with you wearing your baby doll nightie, the minute he walks through the door when it's 'the right time'. Added to this heady brew is the person who is telling you that you are 'trying too hard' and that 'if you only relax, it will happen'. It's a recipe for disaster.

I've had many people weeping at the other end of the phone because 'it hasn't happened'. Frequently, when I ask how long they have been trying, they say something like 'two months', with a big sigh. As you now know, it is usual for it to take quite a bit longer. Let's now tackle the other myths.

Conception is supposed to be good fun, not a dreary

chore. It's the time in your life when you can be completely abandoned in your lovemaking and when you can feel a very special closeness with your partner, and I strongly advise not wrecking it with frequent temperature taking and the like. Accept that it's going to take six months, maybe more, and just enjoy it. And accept that if you are not pregnant after a month or so, there is nothing wrong with you. You are almost certainly horribly normal.

Temperature charts may seem like a novelty for a month, but that soon wears off. The idea is that the body temperature rises slightly after ovulation and you will need to take your temperature not only every morning at the same time, before eating or drinking (a good swig of tea immediately before the thermometer came round was always the way to wangle an extra day in sick bay in my youth), but also be meticulous about recording the result. You can use an ordinary clinical thermometer (Feverscan types are not suitable) obtained from any chemist. The trouble with this palaver is that it isn't very accurate, and it is disruptive. Many women who can show no discernible rise in temperature are ovulating perfectly normally; besides, the temperature change occurs after ovulation, when you really want to be making love before ovulation occurs (since sperm survive longer in the genital tract than the egg). If you must, play around with a thermometer for a month, but then throw it away as being completely useless.

Besides being incredibly expensive, ovulation detection kits are also somewhat suspect in my view. The kits measure the hormone luteinising hormone (LH) which is the signal for the ovary to release an egg. Many women find them confusing to use and, if they have miscalculated the approximate time that they will be ovulating, alarming when they do not register the required colour change. Also, a bit like temperature testing, the results of such tests tend to make women far more despairing, I think, when they don't get pregnant following a cycle in which they've used them.

The truth is that even if you are ovulating, even if your partner has sperm that race away like Linford Christie off the blocks, and even if sperm and egg crash head on *and* the earth moves, you still have only a 1 in 4 chance of getting pregnant in any one cycle. And that's normal. But somehow if you know you've ovulated in a particular month, you expect a result all the more. For the vast majority of couples ovulation detection kits and thermometers are simply not necessary and can put an unwarranted strain on your lovemaking.

It is true that you are more likely to get pregnant if you make love during your fertile period, especially just before ovulation occurs. The way you calculate your fertile period is this: the length of the second half of the cycle is fairly constant, at about 14 days. Keep a record of a few of your cycles. If your shortest cycle was 27 days and your longest 32 (such minor variation in cycle length is well within the normal range), then ovulation is likely to occur in the present cycle between day 13 (27–14) and day 18 (32–14). Based on this, your fertile period is likely to occur somewhere between day 12 and day 19. Making love every couple of days during this time should easily supply enough fertile sperm to do the deed.

Ah, you say, but why did they tell us that we could get pregnant at any time of our cycle when we were at school? In theory, if you had a very short cycle (and teenagers sometimes do) and ovulated early enough, and based on the fact that sperm can loiter for three days or more in the genital tract, you could make love on the last day of your period and get pregnant. You are also at your most fertile as a teenager. There seems to be a time window in which successful conception occurs, and whilst some of us have discrete little windows of no more than twenty-four hours or so, others (who unfairly always live next to an infertile couple) seem to have gaping great patio doors. Unfortunately we do not come with external indicators of fertility, which is, I believe, a serious design fault on the part of our Maker.

Another of these myths is that having sex too often reduces the 'strength' of sperm. In fact, long term abstention reduces sperm quality (monks apparently make very poor sperm donors). Making love every two or three days keeps semen in tip-top condition. Another myth is that you have to have an orgasm in order for pregnancy to occur. Although an orgasm does tend to act as a sort of sperm hoover, sucking sperm up during the womb's contractions, it is not necessary for conception. Artificial insemination wouldn't work if such a thing were true.

You don't have to lie down afterwards, either. I was often asked this by women, and I would always reply by asking them if it were true that you couldn't get pregnant if you did it standing up. 'Old wives' tale,' they said. 'Then you know the answer to your question,' said I. Think about it. Of course semen will run out of the vagina; but this is because semen, having been rather jelly-like ('wallpaper paste' was how one lady described it to me), liquefies after 20–30 minutes. This is long after the special boat squadron of the sperm world are up and at it, and preventing semen running out by lying with your legs up in the air will do nothing for you, apart from being a rather relaxing way to spend a post-coital half hour. The final question concerns position. Does doing it doggy style make it better for women with retroverted – i.e. backward rather than forward tilting – wombs (who are as fertile as everyone else, by the way)? Is adopting a position where deep penetration is more likely better, etc.? The short answer is that you can do it any way you like and it won't make any difference to anything except how much you enjoy that particular session of lovemaking.

As a counsellor, I was often contacted by women – let's call them Filofax conceivers – who had worked out their exact moment of ovulation (not to mention the phase of the moon, the date of the school year, tax year, etc.) and who were making love just once a month convinced that, because they had the 'right moments' sewn up, they would automatically have the greatest possible chance of conception. Real life isn't like this. If you only make love once a month, even if the moon is in Aquarius and you know you are ovulating, you only have a 4 per cent chance of conception in any one cycle. The moral is, the more times you make love the more likely you are to get pregnant. When people ask me, in all seriousness, what I would recommend to ensure pregnancy, my answer is always much simpler than they were expecting – frequent sex. It does the trick nine times out of ten, and that's a guarantee.

When should you seek help? It depends on your age and your symptoms. If you are under 30, it is probably reasonable to wait 18 months to 2 years before embarking on tests. After the age of 30, I would say that you should consult someone if you do not get pregnant within a year, but of course the older you are the more likely it is to take longer. There are some situations in which you should not wait but seek help fairly quickly. These include problems with periods (no periods for some time or very infrequent periods, both of which might indicate ovulation difficulties), recent very heavy periods (possible problems with the womb lining), painful sex and heavy/painful periods (possible endometriosis), or a history of pelvic infection or burst appendix (possible tubal damage). On the male side, undescended testitle, mumps in adult life and testicular damage, injury or surgery should also prompt early attention from an expert.

Secondary infertility can be particularly frustrating. This is when a previous child has been conceived without any problem, but conception of a second child proves difficult. One of the most obvious answers is a change of partner. Fertility is a sum of parts, as you might say, and just because a woman is fertile with one partner does not necessarily mean that she will be as fertile with another partner, even though he too may have had no problems fathering children in a previous relationship. Secondary infertility occurring with the same partner is particularly frustrating, especially if nothing seems to have changed (i.e. periods still the same, no intervening pelvic infection, etc.). Part of it may simply be the effect of passing years and increasing age. In about a third of couples seeking help with infertility, the woman has had a previous child. Here the news is good, and more than 90 per cent of these women become pregnant, although it can take time.

Are there any self-help measures that you can take? There are, as outlined in Chapter 1, but they come with a warning because they are general health measures which, although they may help fertility, will obviously do nothing for you if the cause of your infertility is a blocked tube. I don't want you to believe that just because you are a health fiend, it will guarantee your fertility, because it won't.

As I have said, both partners should give up smoking and cut down on drinking. Heavy drinking certainly causes sperm count to fall in men, and recreational drugs, particularly cannabis, are also known to affect sperm quality. As for men wearing boxer shorts and having cold baths to restore their sperm count, the science to back this one is a bit thin on the ground, although at least one can say that it is something positive, which costs you nothing and isn't harmful. Mind you, a lorry driver's wife interrupted me as I was saying this one day at a WI meeting to say that she had sent her husband off to work each day with a series of ice packs in a coolbox, which she made him sit on during his trips up the M1, to make sure that he kept his scrotum at the required temperature. 'And I got pregnant,' she said proudly. This admission has haunted me ever since, and at motorway service stations I always mentally check every lorry driver for hidden ice packs.

Finally, what of stress? As I indicated earlier, there is always a wise guy (it's usually your mother-in-law) doing the 'it would all be fine if you just relaxed' bit. Having gone through this myself, I know just how – well, stressful – it is to have this sort of thing hurled at you all the time.

Following major burns, levels of the stress hormone cortisol rise enormously, and this is known to affect fertility temporarily in men. Case proved? You might think that to have very little or no cortisol around would be a 'good thing' as far as women were concerned. Curiously, however, recent research has revealed that the presence of cortisol is essential to fertilisation and that nurse cells (the cells that surround and nurture the developing egg) that contain an enzyme that destroys cortisol are indicative of an egg that is unlikely to fertilise.

Our periods are the visible barometer of the effect of stress on our reproductive health, and severe stress, such as final exams, the break-up of a relationship, bereavement, etc., can manifest itself in missed or irregular periods. We are all aware of this, so when people say that stress is the cause of infertility we tend to concur, falling back on our own experiences, and also that hoary old chestnut of the infertile couple who adopt only to conceive immediately themselves. Case proved? I think not.

It is quite normal for fertile women to fail to ovulate occasionally – it's just part of life's rich reproductive tapestry. So what are the facts? Despite the extreme stress of war, poverty and other hardships, women still conceive, and it is apparent that stress is a consequence of infertility rather than its cause. Stress tends to be cited as a cause when other causes are not apparent, but careful evaluation of 'unexplained infertility' shows there to be a demonstrable physical cause or causes in virtually all cases. True psychological causes of infertility are very rare, accounting for less than 2 per cent of all infertility, and even in these cases tend to be psychosexual in origin. Having said all of this, all infertility specialists have seen couples who have decided to give up trying for a bit and have a holiday, only to return pregnant. As for the infertile couple and adoption, the instances are obviously there, but far rarer than popular legend would suggest.

Choosing the Sex of Your Baby

I remember doing a feature on this for *Practical Parenting* many years ago. It was called 'First tie up your left testicle', and it was the subject of more requests for radio and TV interviews than almost anything else I have ever done. Everyone says it's silly but everyone wants to know. So, because this is a book about real pregnancy and the real questions that women ask, here is something on choosing the sex of your baby.

First, how to have a girl . . . For this exercise, you need a squeezy bottle, well washed, two tablespoons of wine vinegar (not malt like the sort that you put on chips) and a pint of water (although Perrier might be more fun, I'd stick to boiled British tap). Mix the vinegar with the water, put it in the squeezy bottle, and put the bottle by the bed, ready for THE moment – well, fifteen minutes before THE moment, actually. If it is between day 7 and day 10 of your cycle, and definitely before the time you ovulate, you may now proceed, having first had a quick sloosh of a douche with the contents of the squeezy bottle. Face-to-face sex is advised, and there must be absolutely no sex after ejaculation. And one other thing, you may not have an orgasm. Oh, didn't I mention that before? Never mind, better luck next month.

And now for the boy . . . Now here, no sex please until ovulation has occurred. It's 5 g of baking soda and a pint of water in the old squeezy bottle this time and, so that you are in the picture early on, female orgasm is permissible, but there is a catch; it must be before the man has ejaculated. This time, the position to be adopted is with the man behind and the women in front, and the procedure must be repeated – omitting nothing – at least three times in the next twenty-four hours.

When women asked me about choosing the sex of their babies, I would tell them this rigmarole, and if they were giggling by the end of it I knew they had taken the advice in the spirit in which it was given. This method of sex selection comes from two American doctors, now discredited, who did rather well out of it for a long time. One wonders how many of their patients actually followed this regime, which seems to me like a fine way to wreck a good sex life. By the way, if the theory behind this were true, and it is very suspect indeed, women who were artificially inseminated at the time of ovulation would all have boys – and they don't. Curiously there is some research which indicates that hormonal environment at the time of conception is an influence. Researchers concluded that more boys were conceived on days 1, 2 and 3 of the fertile period, while more girls were conceived at ovulation – absolutely the opposite of what Shettles, the American who came up with these theories, suggested.

There are statistics to show how the ratio of boys conceived falls during the first year of marriage. There's a well-known saying: 'Sex in marriage is like a medicine. Take it three times a day for the first week, then once a day for another week, then every three or four days until the condition has cleared up.' There is a decline in the ratio of boys conceived as the first year of marriage progresses. Later births are more likely to be female. More frequent sex, researchers assumed, probably meant fertilisation earlier during the three-day period. Frequent sex may also account for the preponderance of boys born after wars.

The possibilities of choosing sex come about because, in effect, the man determines the sex of a baby by providing either an X chromosome or a Y chromosome to pair with the X chromosome provided by the woman's egg. And the thought that you might be able to select the sex of the baby by giving sperm the right conditions has inspired much lunacy, of which the squeezy bottle is but one example. Deep penetration is supposed to give the Y-bearing sperm, which are supposed to be slightly faster swimmers, a head start, and there was some talk that centrifuging sperm, making the slightly heavier, Y-bearing sperm sink, and then inseminating women who wanted boys with just this fraction, would work. You could try this method at home – those salad driers are quite effective centrifuges; but it's not recommended, especially as there is no evidence that it works. Actually, here again I was caught out. A woman phoned me one day, and I told her about this. She rang again the next day. 'Remember me,' she said. 'The salad drier.' How could I have forgotten her? 'Well,' she said, 'you never said to put it in a container first.' Good grief.

Wanting to choose the sex of your baby is not new. Both the ancient Greeks and the French in the early fifteenth century were at it, from the evidence of contemporary documents. The Greeks advocated tying up the left testicle with string, or even cutting the left one off altogether, for men desperate for male heirs; this because the ancient Greeks declared that the site of male sperm production was in the right testicle. This theory is exploded by the fact that one-testicled men produce both boys and girls.

And then there is the pre-conception diet. A couple of French doctors made a great deal of money with a book called *Choosing your Child through your Diet*, published in 1984. It is based on the belief that a diet for the potential mother rich in calcium favours girls and that a diet with a high salt content favours the conception of boys. Here is a quick sample: For girls it is Evian mineral water, and laying off the tea and coffee, with absolutely no alcohol. For boys it is Vichy St Yorre water (rich in the right salts) and lots of beer and cider. As to dairy food, up to 2 litres (yes, 2 litres – that's nearly 4 pints) of milk a day are stipulated in the girl diet, together with yoghurt, unsalted butter and lots of other dairy produce. Boy dieters get to feast on smoked salmon (highly recommended), together with meat, fresh fish and all types of fruit (the girl dieters are only allowed to choose between apples, pears, kiwi fruit and clementines). As far as veg are concerned, boy dieters can eat anything except dandelion leaves (the authors were French, remember). They also suggest that girl dieters eat only minimal quantities of meat 'simmered in water', together with lots of eggs. Funnily enough they reported a huge success with boys – are you surprised, given the girl diet?

These diets have to be started at least two months prior to conception. Since, as you saw earlier in this chapter, the average British couple takes at least six months to conceive, you could be knocking back milk for a very long time. In all seriousness, these diets are highly unbalanced and not what you should be eating prior to conception. Also you'd end up with high blood pressure on the boy diet and either kidney stones or the physique of a Sumo wrestler on the girl diet.

Enough of the hocus pocus. What does science have to

offer? In a variation on the salad-drier technique, various gender clinics have been set up by doctors claiming, by a process of centrifuging and sperm separation, to have achieved 80 per cent success rates. Their methods have not been subject to scientific scrutiny and no one has been able to reproduce them. This is suspicious in itself, although I suppose that the proponents would argue that if they published every Dr Tom, Dick and Harry would be at it too, and presumably they want to keep this money-making wheeze to themselves.

One rather more promising area relates to hormones. It is said that the hormone levels of both parents at the time of conception influence the sex of the child conceived. Hormone levels can be affected by, among other things, diet, stress and disease. For instance people in alcohol-related jobs, such as publicans, have between 6 and 10 per cent more girls than boys. Alcohol reduced the levels of the male hormone testosterone in men, and this could be responsible. On the other hand, butchers have 21 per cent more boys than girls according to a study of 1,220 butchers in the early 1980s. Researchers put this down to the effects of male growth hormones fed to animals, suggesting that the very low levels of hormones still present in the meat – of which butchers, of course, eat an above average amount – could act as a trigger for production of testosterone in the prospective father. In the 1960s and 1970s when cattle were fed oestrogens, butchers had more daughters.

Stress is thought to produce offspring of the opposite sex to the stressed parent. Stress has been shown to lower the levels of the female hormone gonadotrophin in women and of male hormones in men. Wives of men in high-stress jobs – fighter pilots, astronauts and abalone drivers in Australia (don't ask me why abalone diving is stressful) – are known to have more girls than boys. Deep sea divers and anaesthetists are said to beget more girls. When I was doing a television piece about this, we cut to a regional presenter for his opinion. Unknown to me (but known to every other member of the universe) the presenter had donned full deep sea diving kit, complete with an artfully placed piece of seaweed. I then had to keep a straight face while I talked about the science of sex selection. I failed.

Following a recent discovery that individuals can be genetically female, but biologically male, some scientists feel that although gender is determined by an individual's sexual blueprint, it is conditions in the womb at the time that the sex gene is switched on that truly determines sex. Because of circulating female hormones, all babies would be girls, no matter what their chromosomes said – if you like, girls are the default mode – but for this switching device which ensures that at a set moment the fetal testes start to produce male hormones which induce the formation of the penis and other male structures.

The most persuasive studies supporting this theory are of species that produce litters of many young from each pregnancy. During such pregnancies, the babies are arranged like peas in a pod. This grouping results in babies of opposite sex residing next to one another in random order. If this theory is correct, hormones produced by one baby's sex organs could profoundly influence the sex structures in an adjacent baby. This turns out to be true – female babies with male babies on either side are exposed to more testosterone and as a result are more aggressive and less attractive to males than babies with no males on either side. The opposite feminising effect is seen with male babies surrounded by girls. All sorts of questions are raised by this research. Does, for instance, stress during pregnancy, particularly at the time of this gender switching, result in more aggressive children, because of raised testosterone levels?

In truth, there is only one way to select the sex of babies and that is to sex embryos following IVF. Such procedures, pioneered by Professor Robert Winston, have made it possible for couples living in the shadow of genetically determined sex-linked diseases, such as some types of muscular dystrophy, to know right from the start of the pregnancy that their baby will not be affected by this disease.

If you still want sex selection, here are some random thoughts. If going to a war zone (for boys) fails, you could try making love in the spring (boys again) or even, and this one sounds fun, exhausting your partner with frequent love making (with condom attached) and then locking him in the broom cupboard (exhausted sex drive results in more boys). As for girls, try hijacking an anaesthetist for a night of passion behind his gas canisters. I suspect that if I switched my recipes for girls and boys the result would be the same; because for every two couples who want the recipe, the law of averages says that one of them must have a success story to tell me.

3

The First Weeks of Pregnancy

Confirming Pregnancy

So how do you know when you're pregnant? Some women claim to know instantly and may even experience pain on one side of the lower abdomen in the week after conception, which is said to be the fertilised egg travelling down the fallopian tube. For others, symptoms of pregnancy start even before they have missed a period. Extreme tiredness, nausea, a metallic taste in the mouth, tingling boobs, rushing off for a pee every five minutes, or sometimes an aversion to the point of nausea from something you formerly liked a great deal, like red wine, coffee or tea. However, yet more women are completely confused by symptoms of pregnancy – and remember, many of these can be explained a million different ways. For instance, many women find that their breasts tingle or are uncomfortably heavy just before a period – so is this pregnancy, or just a late period? And if you either really want, or really don't want to be pregnant, there is no doubt that you can think yourself into some of these symptoms given a little bit of effort from a fevered imagination.

It's no good torturing yourself. Get down to the chemist and sort yourself out a pregnancy test kit. Although they are quite expensive, they are pretty accurate (they claim 99 per cent, but that is under laboratory conditions, which I have yet to come across in anybody's home – especially at 5 a.m. in a dither of nerves, excitement and anticipation). These tests can be used from the day your period was due. Although most of them say that you can use them at any time of day, it is best to use a urine sample from your first pee of the day because this will have the greatest concentration of the hormone for which the test is sensitive (human chorionic gonadotrophin). The tests vary in how they display results, how long they take, etc., but most will now give a result in five minutes. The test is unaffected by medicines, painkillers or even the contraceptive pill. Positive results are unlikely to be wrong. If you have a weakly positive result, which is then followed by your period within a few days, it indicates that the fertilised egg has failed to implant properly. This is not something to worry about, since research shows that about 70 per cent of conceptions will fail. It does not indicate that you have done anything wrong, simply that this time pregnancy is not to be. You have an excellent chance of conceiving again. A negative result should be repeated three days later to be absolutely sure. Alternatively, you can obtain pregnancy testing free from your GP or family planning clinic. You should take along a sample of your first urine of the day in a clean, well-rinsed container.

You can work out your expected date of confinement by taking the date of your last menstrual period (LMP), adding 7 days and then adding 9 to the month numeral (for instance if your LMP was 2.11.95, adding 7 days will bring you to the 9th, and adding 9 to 11 brings you (and you'll have to use your fingers) to August – so the estimated date of delivery (EDD) is 9.8.96. Only 4 per cent of babies are born on the due date, so this is only a guide.

Even if you very much want to be pregnant, you may find yourself taken by surprise when you get a positive result. You may suddenly think that you don't want a baby after all and feel rather overwhelmed by the enormity of it all – particularly with regard to the practical things: what will the boss say, how are we going to manage, where's the baby going to sleep, the house isn't big enough, etc. If your pregnancy wasn't planned, you may feel completely confused, or even angry – with yourself, with the father of the baby, with the whole world. These feelings are perfectly natural and will usually subside with time. Of course you may want to tell your partner straight away, but whether you do or not, I would then strongly advise sitting on your news for at least a couple of days whilst you both come to terms with it. You may be bursting to tell everyone, particularly if this is your first pregnancy, but some couples, particularly those where there has been a history of miscarriage or other pregnancy problems, prefer not to let anyone know for several months.

You may want to exercise particular caution about telling your boss. In the best of all possible worlds, your caring and enlightened boss will want to think ahead about cover for you during your absence, switching you to projects that perhaps might involve less travel, etc. In practice, some bosses fail to come up to these high ideals and will make decisions for you without consultation, usually with a sharp eye to the balance book rather than your future. Perhaps I am being overly cynical. You certainly don't have to tell him or her straight away – you need to give only twenty-one weeks of notice (i.e. when you are about six months pregnant), with an accompanying maternity certificate which you can obtain from your GP or midwife. However, there should be no loss of pay for keeping antenatal appointments, and obviously you can't have this benefit if you don't tell your employer. You should also tell your employer immediately if you work with hazardous materials such as radiation or chemicals, as there is a statutory obligation on them to move you to another type of work.

One person that you should tell is your doctor. The earlier

you start your antenatal care the better. However, some doctors still take the attitude that there is little they can do in the first three months and you may find, having proudly announced your pregnancy, that you are ignored medically for three months or so. Don't worry about this unduly. You've done the right thing in getting yourself into the system early – now let it catch up with you whilst you do some thinking and some homework.

Where to Have Your Baby

There is usually a bit of form filling required at your first doctor's visit which will entitle you to free dental treatment, prescriptions, etc. Now is the time to start thinking about where to have your baby. You may have firm views already. You may not have made any decisions yet and want to talk to as many people as possible. Don't be surprised if personalities rather than facilities decide your eventual preference. One of the keys to a happy pregnancy and delivery is to be with someone you know and trust – it might be a hospital consultant, it might be a midwife, or the GP you have known all your life. But stick with your instincts and if, having made a choice, you don't like your carer, remember you can always change.

You should have a choice between hospital, a community or GP midwife unit, or home, and this choice will also decide where you have most of your antenatal care. GP units are not that common and the more usual system is one of shared care, whereby your GP or community midwife looks after you for most of the pregnancy (with occasional visits to hospital for scans, etc.) with delivery in hospital. One of the better known arrangements is called DOMINO, which stands for domiciliary in and out: basically your midwife comes to you when labour starts and then takes you to hospital to deliver your baby. There is considerable variation in provision across the country, and if you are new to an area you will be able to get information on what's available locally from your Community Health Council (you will find them listed in the telephone directory).

There may only be one hospital in your area, but in some places, particularly large conurbations, there may be several. In theory you have a right to attend the hospital of your choice as a maternity patient. If a hospital delivery is what you want, then ask other mothers, or your local NCT group, about the pros and cons of each of the hospitals in your area. You may want to take into consideration the quality and friendliness of the medical staff, hospital surroundings or facilities (do they have birthing rooms, is there twenty-four-hour cover by obstetric anaesthetists for epidurals, etc.) or a hospital's policy (for instance, what are their policies about episiotomies or keeping mothers with babies after birth). Another question to ask of a hospital is whether they run a team midwifery scheme (this is where a woman is cared for by a small team of midwives, all of whom will become familiar to her during pregnancy and one of whom will deliver her).

Unless you have a difficult pregnancy or labour, although you are theoretically under the care of a named consultant obstetrician, in practice you are unlikely to see him, which is where team midwifery can make such a difference. It helps enormously to know the people who are delivering you. I confidently say 'him' because there are very few female consultant obstetricians. Many women train in obstetrics but sadly the career structure is such that breaks to have a family pretty much spell the end to a woman's aspirations of becoming a consultant. However, if you would particularly like a woman to deliver you, there are usually at least some women doctors, usually registrars. There are a host of other questions that you may want to ask – such as what is the normal length of stay, or are fathers ever asked to leave the delivery room. The best thing to do in the early months of pregnancy is to keep a notebook in which you write down all the questions that come to you – then you can make sure that each gets answered when you go to the hospital for your first visit.

In our survey, 90 per cent of respondents were delivered in hospital, 6 per cent in GP units, and just under 3 per cent overall at home. There are many arguments for and against home birth which are outside the scope of this book. My personal opinion is that home delivery is less dangerous than it is sometimes made out to be; that being in your own surroundings can help immeasurably, and I have no doubt that it can be a wonderful experience (although certainly not pain free). However, home delivery is emphatically not for everyone. I would personally never encourage someone having a first baby to have it at home – partly because until you have had a baby you have no track record, as it were. What was particularly noteworthy from our survey was that of first time mothers, only 1 per cent had a home delivery, whereas 13 per cent had the fourth child at home. If you want a home birth, you really need specialist information. There are a number of good books on home birth, which address not only the practicalities but also how to go about getting a home birth – something which can be notoriously difficult. Organisations such as AIMS (Association for Improvements in the Maternity Services) can advise you and there are also a number of companies such as Aqua Birth Pools which hire birthing pools, etc., for home use (their addresses are given in Appendix I).

Finally some thoughts on relationships with your carers now that you are pregnant. Part of the problem between carers and pregnant women is that pregnant women are pregnant. This is not to excuse the behaviour of some medical staff who can fall woefully short of the ideal when caring for pregnant women; however, remarks which you wouldn't think twice about if you weren't so emotionally vulnerable can induce fury, or floods of tears, or acute anxiety, or sometimes all three at once. The trouble is that very often pregnant women accept what they are told in silence, do not challenge it at the time and then spend weeks worrying about something which was really nothing. From the survey, it was clear that thoughtless remarks which had no medical import were often taken to heart, and were the subject of great unhappiness which could easily have been resolved. My second baby was still in the breech position – i.e. bottom down instead of head down, at the thirty-four weeks, and a midwife said casually, talking to the baby, 'You'd better turn round in there or it's the knife for your mum.' Although she was being light-hearted, and although I know perfectly well that second and subsequent babies, in particular, frequently turn late, it didn't stop me from getting into a complete panic. If I had said, 'But won't the baby turn round?' I'm sure I would have got the reassurance I needed. But I was just so overwhelmed that I said something cheery, slid off into the night and never asked (and the blighter did turn around). So my first rule of pregnancy is to ask, ask and ask again until you are satisfied that you understand and that you have the information you need.

My second rule is not to set your heart on having things a particular way. We all hope that pregnancy will proceed without any hitch at all. And this may be exactly what happens to you. But if you are too wedded to the romance of pregnancy, real life may rudely intervene, particularly if you have later pregnancy problems such as pre-eclampsia (see Chapter 11) which may require an early admission to hospital. Not at all what you had planned. It's hard when it doesn't happen the way you want – particularly if all your friends seemed to sail through pregnancy – and you can feel very disappointed, cheated and demoralised. But at the end of the day, pregnancy occupies a very short time in your life; you have the rest of your life to spend with that baby, and that is what you may have to keep telling yourself. So approach your pregnancy with a completely open mind, and whatever you do, don't decide how it's going to be the minute the test says positive.

The third rule of pregnancy is about partnerships – not with your best loved, but with your carers. If you can, and this is where schemes where you see the same person pretty much all the way through have such an advantage, try hard to strike up a relationship with your carer, one in which you approach pregnancy and birth as partners on a united front. Sometimes this can be incredibly difficult. Some carers can be aloof, or patronising, but most would not be in this line of work if they did not enjoy the company of women or if they were not still excited by the birth process and what it means for those they care for. You have to work hard at it sometimes, but the return is handsome. Communicate with your carer, and most times you'll get a lot back. And remember, if you cannot forge a relationship, or actively dislike your carer, you really can change – go to a hospital if you don't like your GP, ask for a different midwife, and – what many people don't realise – ask if you can change a consultant for another one; such requests are normally sympathetically received.

Going to Hospital

Allow yourself hours for your visit to hospital, and take a good book – I suggest something racy and distracting. Hospitals vary enormously in the timing of their 'booking visit', some offer them as early as 8 weeks, whilst others leave it to 18 weeks. There will be a great deal of 'history taking'. You will be asked about previous pregnancies, about previous births, if applicable, and about your concerns for this pregnancy. There will be a detailed family and personal history – on the lines of, have you ever had heart disease, diabetes, etc., etc., what operations have you had, and so on. You will be asked your ethnic origin. The answers to these questions will give your carers clues as to how this pregnancy might progress, and whether you need further care. For instance, if your ethnic origin is African, you might be a carrier for sickle cell disease and might therefore require specialist antenatal testing. A family history of diabetes might indicate that you are at greater risk of problems affecting sugar metabolism during your pregnancy, previous surgery may indicate whether or not you tolerate anaesthesia well and reveal a condition of relevance to this pregnancy. In other words, this is an attempt to pigeonhole you in an appropriate risk box. However, risk scoring is not a very effective predictor of outcome with only 10–30 per cent of women experiencing the adverse outcome for which the scoring system declares them at risk – something you need to remember when 'high risk' is being slapped on your notes.

The position with medical records is changing all the time. Most pregnant women now have a 'co-operation card' which has all the basic details about your current pregnancy, so that you can hand it to your carer if for any reason you need to be admitted to another hospital (whilst on holiday or away from home, for instance) – but nobody will now object if you want to look at your own notes. It is probable that you have an entirely open relationship with your partner, but you may not have wanted to tell him about a previous pregnancy or termination. Be aware that your notes, which will hang about the place during labour, will reveal this. There is a section which will say 'Parity': if you have no children but have had one previous termination, you will see Para 0 + 1 (TOP) or Grav (gravity) 2 (TOP) where TOP stands for termination of pregnancy. If this is a concern to you, tell the midwife taking your notes. Your co-op card will only have details of your current pregnancy.

The booking visit is the time to ask all those questions you have by now written down in that notebook – so have them ready.

At this visit, you will have your height measured. This will give an indication as to the size of your pelvis. Women used also to be asked to provide their shoe size, because it was thought that a disproportionate shoe size to height might indicate someone who was at risk of pelvic disproportion. Although it is true that small women are more likely to have caesarean sections, there is no real science behind this, and shoe size is no long requested. You will be asked for a sample of blood and this will be typed (i.e. your blood group will be determined) and your rubella status and antibody level assessed. Some hospitals may also do anonymised HIV testing, and most hospitals still undertake Wasserman testing on all blood – this is a test for syphilis which, although now a very rare disease, poses such grave dangers for the baby that testing can still be justified. Most hospitals also test for hepatitis B. Additional testing may be appropriate depending on your ethnic group. Your haemoglobin levels will be measured, as a low haemoglobin level indicates anaemia, which will need to be treated. You are likely to have a further blood test at 28 weeks, and at 36 weeks when your antibody and haemoglobin levels will be rechecked. Women whose blood group is rhesus negative may have more frequent blood testing.

You will be given a general medical examination, with a doctor listening to your heart and lungs. Pregnancy puts a particular strain on both. It is not uncommon for heart murmurs to be discovered. In most women, this is a variation of normal which is of no significance and which will not affect outcome of pregnancy, but which nevertheless may prompt further investigation from a cardiologist, just to be sure. Your tummy will be subjected to some prodding (the technical term is palpation) and at later hospital visits the height of your fundus will be assessed. I love this phrase, height of the fundus – it sounds so impressive. All it actually means is that the position of the top of your womb (the fundus) which is pushed ever upwards during pregnancy, is charted and then compared to the average fundal height for a woman of the same gestation as you. If there is a discrepancy, then further investigation, usually ultrasound, will be suggested. The most likely reason for discrepancy is that you have your dates wrong.

A note will also be made, at later visits, of how your baby is lying. At its most basic, you will find vertex or cephalic (abbreviated to Vx or C) meaning head down, transverse (lying crossways), or breech (bottom down). At later stages of pregnancy, a note will be made of your baby's position. Again, there are a series of abbreviations, for instance LOA means left occiput anterior – your baby's head is on your left side with the occiput bone (the back of the head) frontwards; that is, your baby is facing your backbone. ROP would mean that your baby's head is on your right, the occiput bone facing backwards so that the baby is facing forward.

In the early months of pregnancy, when fundal height is more difficult to assess, the doctor may estimate the stage of your pregnancy by putting two fingers inside your vagina, whilst palpating the abdomen. This approach also allows the doctor to check you for the presence of things like ovarian cysts and fibroids. Again, it is quite common for a cyst to be detected – most are the sort that hang over after an egg has been released from a follicle and will resolve by themselves. However, unusually, they can be a source of pain, and it is as well that your carers know about your cyst as otherwise there is a risk that abdominal pain may be wrongly diagnosed. Some hospitals may not undertake any vaginal examinations, preferring to rely completely on ultrasound scanning.

At this and all subsequent visits you will be weighed, your blood pressure will be checked because of concern about pre-eclampsia (see Chapter 11) and your urine will be tested for the presence of protein and sugar.

MEASURING WEIGHT GAIN

Pregnancy manuals tend to show nice little weight charts, where weight is put on at a uniform rate over the pregnancy. Any woman who has been pregnant will tell you that it doesn't work like this. Weight is put on in fits and starts, and there may be a point in pregnancy (usually about 20–24 weeks) when you wake up one morning to discover that it looks as if someone had crept behind you in the night with a football pump, so noticeable has your bulge suddenly become. There is a lot of confusion about weight gain in pregnancy and pregnancy books used to be very severe – no more than 8 to 9 kg is Gordon Bourne's suggestion in *Pregnancy*, Pan, 1996. Bourne goes so far as to say that obstetricians associate an excessive weight gain with pre-eclapsia. In fact, this is the cart pulling the horse because it is pre-eclampsia which causes the fluid retention which results in weight gain.

Nevertheless, swelling accompanied by a rapid weight gain – over 1 kg (2.2 lbs) a week for more than two or three weeks, should ring warning bells. If you are retaining fluid, you may be told to restrict your fluid intake as this is 'causing the problem'. This is tosh. What you drink will not affect whether fluid is retained or not – the problem is that your blood vessels are leaky (see Chapter 11), not that you are drinking too much.

MEASURING BLOOD PRESSURE

Blood pressure is not constant. It alters, not just from day to day, but from one minute to the next, according to whether you are resting, sleeping or exercising, and even according to whether you are standing up or sitting down. It also alters with age, so that a blood pressure reading which might cause concern in pregnancy would be normal for an older woman.

In order to understand how a reading is presented, bear in mind that the pressure of the blood within the arteries rises and falls with each heartbeat – the highest pressure, the systolic, is achieved when the heart beats and the lowest pressure, the diastolic, is recorded when the heart relaxes between beats. When blood pressure is noted, the systolic pressure figure appears over the top of the diastolic one. Thus a blood pressure of 110/70 means a systolic of 110 mmHg (millimetres of mercury – the measure of blood pressure) and a diastolic of 70 mmHg. Doctors are more concerned by the diastolic reading, – the bottom one – because it is less likely to be affected by the stress of the moment.

From what I have just said, and from the word that is used for consistently raised blood pressure – hypertension – you might think that raised blood pressure has a great deal to do with stress. Of course stress, as in the overworked, jet-setting executive, can play a part; indeed, the phenomenon by which blood pressure rises in response to being measured (so-called 'white coat' syndrome) is a classic example of stress affecting blood pressure. Pregnancy is very often beset with stressful life events – why, for instance, do women get an insane urge to move house when pregnant? – and the conditions in which most women are forced to compete for attention in antenatal clinics is enough to raise anyone's blood pressure. It is perhaps not surprising, therefore, that a woman faced with a high blood pressure reading in pregnancy believes that she is to blame, and that if only she relaxed and 'took things easy' the problem would go away. This is reinforced by the attitude of some unhelpful (and misinformed) medical staff who advise bed rest, and say things like, 'You've been overdoing things, haven't you?' No doubt they mean to be kind.

The truth is this. Any consistent rise in blood pressure in pregnancy (i.e. which is evident despite several readings) is not brought on by working too hard, staying up too late, worrying too much or not putting your feet up enough; neither will it be cured by rest or relaxation. Your body is sending you the clearest possible signal that there is something wrong. You must not ignore this signal, or attempt to explain it away. Professor Chris Redman, an internationally renowned expert on pre-eclampsia, has a very useful analogy. He suggests that you should view a raised blood pressure in the same way as you would a raised temperature. Nobody believes that a temperature is caused by stress or tension, or that you can make it go away by relaxing. A high temperature is a symptom, just like high blood pressure. Only when the cause, perhaps an infection, has gone, will your temperature return to normal. The same is true of your blood pressure – until your baby is delivered, you are likely to continue to experience symptoms.

Many clinics feel that once women have a blood pressure reading of 140/90 mmHg, they should be admited to hospital. In itself, this is not a massive blood pressure and, in the absence of any other symptoms, it may be an indication of underlying chronic hypertension, and not pre-eclampsia at all. If this is the case, there are no direct ill effects on the pregnancy. However, since pre-eclampsia is more common in those who have existing hypertension, blood pressure, urine and weight should continue to be monitored very closely. But the presence of proteinuria, plus a blood pressure reading of 140 over 90, would pretty well ensure hospital admission. Having said that, depending on the degree of proteinuria or other symptoms, hospital admission may be advisable with lower blood pressure readings. There are no absolutes here.

URINE TESTING

Urine is tested for the presence of protein at each antenatal visit, using a commercial dipstick which gives an instant result, recorded as 'trace', +, ++, up to four pluses. 'Trace' may not mean much, if anything, but one plus means that there is definitely something amiss. Incidentally, the test measures concentration of protein rather than the total amount. Thus, if it is a hot day and your urine is quite concentrated you may have an alarming amount of pluses when, if your urine was more dilute, fewer would be recorded. If there is time, the result can be checked by collecting urine over twenty-four hours and measuring the total amount of protein excreted during this time.

Your urine will also be measured for the presence of sugar. During pregnancy, the ability of the body to metabolise sugars alters. After a meal, sugar levels in the blood remain high so that they can be easily transferred across the placenta to the baby. Normally there is no sugar in the urine, but it is common for pregnant women to have some sugar in their urine, particularly if they have recently eaten a heavy meal. If you persistently have sugar in your urine, a glucose tolerance test may be instituted, in which you are asked to drink a measured amount of glucose drink, with various before and after measurements of blood sugar levels. The point of all of this relates to the possibility of diabetes. There are many concerns for women who are diabetic, with the possibility of an overlarge baby (fetal macrosomia) being one of the most pressing.

Just because your body isn't doing its stuff with glucose, however, does not mean that you are going to be diabetic from now on. What you are likely to have is a temporary sort of pregnancy-induced diabetes, called gestational diabetes, or diabetes diagnosed in pregnancy. At one time glucose tolerance tests were almost routine, but there is simply no justification for this, as for a start they are very often wrong (tests have shown that they are not reproducible between 50–70 per cent of times) and falsely labelled many women as having this 'condition'. It remains true that most big babies are born to women with normal glucose tolerance tests, so I would say, be comforted by the fact that you are under surveillance but don't worry about the implications for either you or your baby.

4

Diet during Pregnancy

I include this chapter only to demonstrate that whatever you are eating, some other pregnant woman somewhere is eating sardine and jam sandwiches and loving them every bit as much as you are. The responses in our survey to the question 'Did you have any strange food cravings in pregnancy?' were simply amazing.

Here are just some: 300 ice cubes a day; curried beetroot; chocolate powder on toast; oranges; sucking flannels; chewing elastic bands; olives and mint chocolate biscuits together; peppermint creams and pickled onions together; marmite and banana sandwiches; beetroot and condensed milk sandwiches; sardine and jam sandwiches; kippers with jam on – if you are not feeling sick by now, you should be!

Overall, 17 per cent of women in our survey found that they had cravings for fruit, particularly oranges and lemons. Pickles, as beloved of popular mythology, were a craving for 12 per cent of our respondents. Other favoured foods were ice lollies, ice cream and chocolates.

Women's perception of taste definitely changes during pregnancy. Many pregnant women, for instance, cannot tolerate red wine or coffee during the early months of pregnancy. Quite simply, they taste disgusting. Certainly going off coffee (something I love) was always the best indication of pregnancy in my case. It has been advanced that this is a physiological mechanism which prevents women eating harmful foods in early pregnancy. I am not sure there is evidence to support this, but it's an interesting theory. The point about pregnancy eating is that, whilst you may have cravings for certain foods, they are unlikely to be harmful unless you eat them to the exclusion of all other food. Pica – the technical term for cravings for non-food substances such as coal – was not common among our respondents. One lady said that she ate the fur out of her kettle (something I've come across on a number of occasions), another said that she had taken to sucking bars of soap, but only at night in case her husband discovered what she was doing. Presumably foaming at the mouth would have been a giveaway. Incidentally, don't lay in a supply of kettle fur especially for your next pregnancy – cravings alter from one pregnancy to the next.

To me, one of the most interesting features of this cross-section of dietary preference in pregnancy was the frequency with which chocolates, ice cream, fast food, crisps, fizzy drinks and sweets appeared in the list. I would be failing you if I did not mention what our respondents also said in the 'I wish I'd known' and 'advice' sections. Here are just a few of the hundreds of comments that appeared on the subject of weight gain in pregnancy:

'Don't put on too much weight. I only found out afterwards just how hard it is to lose.'

'By the time I was four months pregnant, I looked like a barrel. Everyone said it was fluid. I knew it wasn't because I just stuffed myself from morning to night and it resulted in me being very uncomfortable. In my next pregnancy, I was much more careful about my weight, and as a result, I had a much more enjoyable pregnancy.'

'Pregnancy was great for me. No more holding my

breath as I went past mirrors and I didn't have a waist, so I indulged myself. I wish I hadn't because now my children are 4 and 2, I'm still trying to lose the weight I put on then.'

'Take a photo of yourself when you were full term. You'll never believe the size you were – and no matter how tubby you are, you'll feel you're thin in comparison.'

'Don't use pregnancy as an excuse to eat everything you want.'

I think this last respondent has got it about right. You will find that you have a ferocious appetite, but don't use it as an excuse; fill the gap with quality snack food: raw fruit, low fat yogurts, etc. – not with fizzy drinks, ice cream and sweets.

I would be doing you a disservice if I included this information in the post-birth section of this book, as by then it is far too late. There is no other way to put it. If you put on a lot of weight during your pregnancy, you will find it very hard to lose afterwards. The most important determinant of your baby's health is your pre-pregnancy weight, not your weight at delivery. Obstetricians used to be very strict about weight gain in pregnancy because of concerns about pre-eclampsia, which was thought at one time to be precipitated by excessive weight gain. It is now known that weight gain (principally because of retained fluid) is a consequence of pre-eclampsia, not its cause. Obstetricians were also concerned about women who did not put on much weight, because low weight gain was linked with a higher risk of prematurity and small-for-dates babies. However, this association is also flawed because small babies weigh less, and have less amniotic fluid, and thus in themselves cause low maternal weight gain.

Incidentally, if you have a baby who is small for dates,

eating more will not make the baby bigger, although rest may be helpful. The problem here is poor transfer of nutrients across the placenta, so that whatever you eat isn't transferred to the baby properly. A very poor diet in pregnancy will result not just in a slightly smaller baby, but will significantly affect your baby's future health. Small babies, with large placentas, are at greater risk of heart disease and diabetes in later life than babies of average size. However, overeating will not result in a noticeably healthier baby, although it may be a bit bigger, but you will be very uncomfortable – so you should be the one concerned about weight gain, not your doctor.

If you are underweight, you should aim to put on no more than 40 lbs; if you are of normal weight for height, no more than 35 lbs, and if you are overweight, no more than 25 lbs. Assuming a 7½ lb baby, it, the fluid and placenta account for no more than 10 lbs in weight.

Interestingly it is thin women who usually put on most weight in pregnancy, because the body is laying down fat stores which were either depleted or absent. If you are short, you should aim to put on slightly less than the maximum as otherwise you may have an excessively large baby which could cause complications during delivery. You should not diet during pregnancy; if you find yourself putting on too much weight then change your eating patterns, cutting out empty calories, and try taking more exercise. Women who stop smoking for pregnancy are particularly vulnerable to rapid weight gain but this is not a reason to continue smoking, merely an indication that you need to be particularly careful about what you eat.

You will find that, when you have your baby, there is an immediate weight loss of about 10 lbs or so, but don't expect miracles in the weight loss department – after all, it took nine months to put on. Your body remains in its energy-efficient mode for a couple of months after delivery and your fat stores may not be fully mobilised (I think this is a sentence you should write down and put on your fridge to comfort yourself) immediately as a result. Breast feeding does mobilise fat stores, especially from the hips and thighs, although only women who are consistent about breast feeding over a long period are likely to lose much weight because of it – a six-week flirtation with breast feeding will do a lot for your baby, but not that much for your fat stores, I am afraid. Some women (about 20 per cent, and I fear I was one of them) lose a good deal of weight very suddenly after birth. But for most women, a realistic expectation would be to be within half a stone of your pre-pregnancy weight by about three months after the birth and within 3 lbs of your normal weight within a year. About 2 per cent of women will increase their weight by 20 lbs or more.

There are lots of reasons why women find it hard to lose weight after delivery. They may not, because they're not feeling up to it, or because there is simply no longer the opportunity, get back to their accustomed level of exercise. They may also find the temptation of being at home, rather than at work all day, with a full fridge, an irresistable excuse to snack. I think by far the best advice, apart from not putting it on in the first place, is to join a postnatal exercise group. It's a good way of meeting other new mums, and there is no doubt about it, trying to lose weight gain en masse with lots of support and encouragement works best for most people. Do be a bit careful, however, about throwing yourself back into exercise. Your ligaments are very soft and vulnerable and I don't think I would advise much beyond some gentle swimming, walking and of course pelvic floor exercises (see Chapter 17) in the first six weeks.

One of the greatest concerns raised by the survey was about information on eating in pregnancy. Pregnant women are a uniquely vulnerable group and almost every diktat on food, from liver to soft cheese, has been aimed at them. It is an immensely confusing area. And you may find it difficult getting advice from your carers partly because they, like you, are probably getting most of their information from the media – the information that they were taught being woefully out of date within just a few years. It is difficult to put some of the scares into perspective; listeriosis, for instance, remains a rare complication of pregnancy affecting only 1 in 20,000 women.

There are three concerns about food: first, that you will acquire some sort of parasitic infection such as toxoplasmosis (see page 27); second that you will catch some sort of food-borne bacterium which will put the baby at risk because of your sickness and fever, for instance salmonella, or because the infection crosses the placenta, e.g. listeria, and third, the more general area, that too much or too little of certain foods will harm your baby. So whilst there are some basic pointers which I can signpost for you, I would strongly recommend that you obtain a copy of *Healthy Eating for You and Your Baby* by Fiona Ford, Robert Fraser and Hilary Dimond (Pan, 1994) which reviews the whole subject very clearly. These authors also run a Nutrition in Pregnancy helpline (see Appendix I), if you have specific concerns.

You should be scrupulous about food hygiene during pregnancy. Wash salads and fruits before consumption. Cook meat thoroughly (or if you want to eat rare meat ensure that it has been deep frozen to $-20°C$ for twenty-four hours before thorough defrosting in the fridge and cooking). Ensure that when you prepare meat you wash your hands, preparation area and utensils carefully afterwards. Separate cooked and raw foods in the fridge, with raw foods on the bottom shelves. Use your nose and eyes to determine whether food is safe for you to eat and ensure that you eat food within the use-by dates. If in doubt when pregnant, don't. Avoid eating high risk foods like meat pies, soft-whip-type ice cream from vans and shell-fish from non-reputable sources. Go for individually packaged portions rather than for portions taken from open bowls or displays. If you are going to reheat food, chill the portions you intend to reheat, and when you are ready to eat it ensure that it is piping hot. Always observe recommended standing times if you are using a microwave and make sure that food is heated to piping hot throughout. An awful lot of this stuff is just common sense for a lifetime's practice.

As far as eggs are concerned, do not eat raw eggs, or foods such as ice cream or mousses that contain them. Shop-bought mayonnaise or salad cream is fine. The other main source of salmonella is poultry; you should therefore be particularly careful to buy your poultry from a reputable source and cook it thoroughly. Listeria is contracted from certain types of cheese, cook-chill foods and pâté. Hard cheese is fine, as is mozzarella and cream cheeses such as Philadelphia, but avoid ripened soft cheese such as Brie and Camembert and blue-veined cheeses such as Stilton, cambozola and Danish blue. Having said this, if you have eaten these cheeses, you shouldn't panic unneces-sarily; listeria remains, as I have indicated, a very rare complication of pregnancy and it is sure and certain that many thousands of women eat such cheeses during pregnancy without coming to any harm. Pâté should not be eaten in pregnancy unless it is bought in individual shrink-wrapped portions with 'pasteurised' on the label. The other concern about pâté is that it is often made from liver, which is not advised during pregnancy because of its high vitamin A content (see page 23). You should not drink unpasteurised milk.

As for eating what your baby needs – that is more difficult. If you're healthy on the diet you eat, then the baby will probably be healthy too. There is absolutely no need to eat for two and you only need the equivalent extra calories of a couple of slices of toast a day, so there really is no excuse! Eat plenty of fruit and vegetables, preferably raw or only lightly cooked. Frozen are sometimes preferable in terms of vitamin content to those wilting, been-at-the-greengrocers-a-week, 'fresh' things. Fruit and vegetables are not only a source of vitamins such as folate, but of fibre which will help prevent constipation. Include starchy foods such as rice, pasta, breakfast cereals and bread in your daily diet which will fill you up without too many calories. Eat some protein every day, such as lean meat, fish or eggs, or alternative sources of protein such as pulses if you are a vegetarian. Dairy foods are a vital source of calcium and should form part of your daily diet too. Try not to eat too many sugary or fatty foods. Women used to be routinely supplemented with iron during pregnancy but it is now known that this isn't necessary, except for women with established anaemia. If you are vegan or vegetarian you should make a special effort to eat iron-containing foods such as bran-fortified cereals, spinach and lentils. Whole grains and soya products reduce iron absorption, as do caffeine-containing drinks, so be aware of this when meal planning. If you are taking iron pills, wash them down with orange or grapefruit juice, as the vitamin C improves absorption.

Fluid intake is important, and although there have been numerous studies on the effect of caffeine during pregnancy, the results have been conflicting. The best advice would be to moderate your coffee and tea drinking and find other drinks instead. However, be careful if you are substituting herbal teas. Some of them are positively dangerous in pregnancy, including feverfew, golden seal, mistletoe, mugwort, penny-royal, rue and tansy. Raspberry leaf tea is sold for use in labour and should not be taken much before this time. If in doubt consult a qualified medical herbalist (there is an address in Appendix I for the organisation which holds a list of registered herbalists), and don't rely on the advice of the girl who takes your money in the health food shop as it is highly likely that she knows less than you.

Alcohol drinking is discussed in detail on page 18 – but you may find yourself wanting to drink, if not much, then a bit, later in pregnancy. Should you or shouldn't you? The recommendation is no more than 8 units a week, with no more than 2 in any one day. There is no evidence that drinking this much or less causes any harm, and I would personally say that if you find that one of the most relaxing parts of your day is when you sit down in the evening, put your feet up and have a small glass of wine, then I wouldn't forsake the benefit of proper relaxation for concern about what one glass might do. My one caveat would be that if you are also smoking, you are increasing the effect of alcohol, and of the two, smoking is the one to give up rather than the odd glass of wine.

5

Antenatal Testing

'Waiting for the result of the amnio was the worst three weeks of my life.'

It wasn't a surprise to learn that nearly 40 per cent of those who completed the survey reported themselves 'very worried' about the health of their baby during pregnancy. Nor was it a surprise to find that in fact, despite this intense anxiety, just 1 in 20 of those surveyed had babies with problems of any kind at birth. You might think that antenatal testing would alleviate some of this worry; if anything, it heightened it. Many hundreds of you reported specific concerns about testing, especially related to triple test. About 10 per cent were very worried about testing, and this was strongly correlated with age – the older the mother, the more likely you were to be anxious about testing. The same proportion, about 10 per cent, had test results that were adverse. This doesn't mean, incidentally, that 10 per cent had babies with a handicap – it means that 10 per cent of results raised question marks about the baby's health which required further investigation.

'I wish I'd known more about testing before I got into it.'

One of the confusions about testing seems to be what the tests are for. If you get a negative result, doesn't this mean that your baby is guaranteed free from handicap? Well, no, it doesn't. Tests are very specific; although they may answer one question, they may leave many others unanswered. It helps if you understand what the tests are looking for and what they can, and can't, tell you.

There are three main groups of handicapping conditions: physical defects, inherited genetic disease and chromosome abnormalities. If you want to find out whether a baby has any physical defects, an ultrasound scan would be appropriate. The baby might appear to be fine, and might indeed have no physical defects at birth, but might still have cystic fibrosis, an inherited genetic disease. The point here is that, by having an ultrasound scan, you were only asking the question, 'Is this baby, as far as we can see, physically normal?' The answer to the question, 'Has this baby got a specific genetic disease?' can only be answered by using a different procedure, such as amniocentesis. The rub is that although amniocentesis might give you the information you require about cystic fibrosis, it won't tell you whether the baby has all ten toes. It's very much horses for courses.

Physical defects are the most common of abnormalities at birth, with heart problems being the most frequent, followed by limb disorders and conditions involving the central nervous system such as spina bifida. Ultrasound is the most appropriate testing procedure, but certain physical defects, like spina bifida, can be diagnosed in other ways, for example through AFP testing and triple test (see page 92).

Inherited gene defects are the next most common group of conditions. Almost all of us carry several inherited gene defects. For instance, 1 in 20 British people carries the gene for cystic fibrosis. But the reason why only 1 in 1,500 babies actually has cystic fibrosis is because we inherit our genes in pairs, and providing we inherit a 'good' copy along with the 'bad', its instructions override that of the 'bad' copy. Carriers of CF do not have the condition and are quite 'normal'. Only if the baby receives a double dose of the bad gene (and both parents would have to be carriers for this to happen) will the baby be affected. This explains why so many people who have a baby with CF have no family history of the disease.

There are about 5,000 so-called single gene defects, with more being documented all the time. Basically they are a small misprint in the genetic instruction manual contained in each cell. Despite the insignificance of the size of the misprint, the meaning of the instruction is altered completely, rather as if someone took down a message incorrectly, putting 'throw out the cat' instead of 'throw out the mat'. Some of these defects can arise as spontaneous mutations – the type of dwarfism called achondroplasia can occur like this – or can be inherited from generation to generation, usually in a set and quite distinctive pattern. About 3 per cent of couples come from families which are affected by genetic disease of one sort or another, and they will need to have genetic counselling, together with very specific testing. This whole field is advancing at a tremendous pace at present and new tests are being developed all the time. If you want to know whether testing is available for a particular condition, you should contact the Genetic Interest Group, an umbrella group of voluntary organisations concerned with genetic disorders. Their address and phone number are in Appendix I. They will also be able to tell you where your nearest regional genetic centre is located.

Most of the tests for gene defects require a sample of the baby's cells. These can be obtained via amniocentesis, CVS or cordocentesis, which are all invasive procedures carrying a risk of miscarriage. This sort of testing wouldn't be carried out unless it was prompted by family history. However, as I have explained, you can be carrying a defective gene and be completely unaware of it, although it is possible now to find out whether you are a cystic fibrosis carrier. The test is easy (it involves rinsing the mouth with a special fluid, which is then spat out), but you are advised to have counselling prior to and after the test. Details can be obtained through the Cystic Fibrosis Trust. There is no point in only one partner having this test, however. Of course, if you test negative for a particular genetic defect you can still have a baby with another type of genetic defect altogether.

The third and final group of handicapping conditions is of those caused by chromosome disorders, which include Down's Syndrome as well as Turner's Syndrome. You will recall that chromosomes are the structures within each cell that carry genetic information. In general, chromosome disorders are not inherited (although there are a few that are). They arise because, either within the sperm or egg or at conception, chromosomes, whilst doing their thing, have become tangled up and haven't done what they should. The analogy I always use is that of having a great heap of green and white spaghetti and trying to sort it out into a white pile and a green pile. You'll find that bits of the green stick onto the white, some bits get broken and some disappear altogether during your sorting efforts.

In general, chromosome disorders are present from conception and will affect only that pregnancy. You can't 'see' gene defects but you can 'see' chromosome disorders, although you need a high-powered microscope to do so. Once again, a sample of the baby's cells is required, which is obtained via amniocentesis, CVS or cordocentesis. The chromosomes are first spread out, then they are identified and put in numerical order (each pair of chromosomes is quite distinct, one from another, and each has a number), from 1–23. This is called karyotyping. From the karyotype, you can tell whether the baby is a girl or a boy and whether there are the right number of chromosomes (thus detecting Down's Syndrome, for instance, which involves an additional chromosome). You can also check that the chromosomes look the right shape and size – are there bits missing, for instance? Although examination of a karyotype should be sufficient to spot major chromosome problems, it might not be sufficient to detect more subtle abnormalities. And karyotyping will not detect a gene defect.

There is some overlap with all of this; for instance, aspects of the baby's physical appearance as seen on ultrasound scan may ring alarm bells as to a potential chromosome problem. Many of these so-called 'soft signs' are not significant in themselves – for instance a bigger gap than normal between the big toe and the next toe might just be, well, a bigger gap. But if the baby were also to have thickened neck folds, plus a number of other signs, it would be highly indicative of Down's Syndrome, although karyotyping would be required before this could be confirmed for sure.

Deciding Whether to Have Testing

'I decided against tests and I'd do the same thing in another pregnancy but I worried terribly about my baby.'

The issue of whether to test or not is one that may be very clearcut for you. If it is, I suspect that you are in the minority. Many women think that they have come to terms with the issues involved in antenatal testing prior to pregnancy, only to find that being pregnant changes their perspective entirely. Pregnancy makes it very hard to think things through with any clarity, yet it is the time when we are forced to make major decisions which have the power to affect not only our own lives but those of our partner and family too. You may feel sure about your decisions one minute, and question them the next – it's part of being pregnant, and quite normal.

You may think that some decisions about testing are relatively easy. For instance, AFP testing is non-invasive, carries no risk to you or your baby, and everyone else seems to be having it. But such tests can have a domino effect, where the discovery of a positive result, in this case a raised AFP level, can lead to much more invasive forms of testing such as amniocentesis. Although you may have previously decided to reject the amnio route, once you have such a potentially serious question mark raised about the health of your baby, there is no turning back – unless you are prepared to endure the remainder of your pregnancy in a state of acute anxiety. As you wait for a test result, you may wish that you had never had testing in the first place. As I said, reassurance is bought at a price.

'My doctor said he wouldn't give me an amniocentesis unless I agreed to have a termination before I had the amnio.'

Many people equate testing with termination, saying that there is no point going ahead with testing if you are not prepared to have a termination in the case of an adverse outcome. I disagree. For me, testing is about information, and I don't believe that you can make any decision about a baby's future in advance of having proper information about its condition. If an ultrasound scan reveals a heart defect, termination is not the only option. It might be, but this is dependent on a whole host of variables which will include, in addition to your own feelings, how severe the problem is and what the prognosis is. There are many heart defects that can now be remedied, although specialist facilities and expertise will be necessary. Prior knowledge of your baby's needs – for instance, the requirement to have the baby in a hospital that has ready access to the necessary type of care, may make the difference between a good and bad outcome.

If, through testing, you discover that your baby has or is likely to have Down's Syndrome, termination does not have to be the option you choose, although some couples may do so. You may prefer to use the information you have gained to prepare yourself and your family for the birth of a baby who will be different to other babies. Unfortunately, only invasive testing with its attendant risk of miscarriage will give you the definitive answer you need.

People who say there is no point in having testing unless you are prepared to terminate the pregnancy make an assumption that test results are always black or white. They are not, and this is something you need to appreciate in advance of testing. For instance, you may have decided that you would indeed terminate a pregnancy affected by Down's Syndrome. You have an amniocentesis, only to discover that although your baby is free of Down's, it has Klinefelter's Syndrome (i.e. is a male baby who has an additional X chromosome). The only 'symptoms' of Klinefelter's may be sterility and scant body hair. There may be a 10–20 point reduction in verbal skills, but performance scores are usually normal and severe retardation uncommon. Now what do you do? Incidentally, if you come across a doctor like the one mentioned by our respondent above, remember that no one can force you to have a termination. If you have to agree to it to get your testing, do so, but you are absolutely free to change your mind at any time.

Of course, you may decide not to have testing at all,

preferring to find out about your baby when he or she is born.
You may reason that 39 out of 40 British babies are normal and
that statistics are on your side – and you'd be right. If this is
your view, you should be supported in it, but you may find
that your friends and family do not share your opinion and
soon the very decision you took to avoid stress and pressure is
causing just that, as your family and friends repeatedly question
the wisdom of your decision. You just have to be courageous
about this, but it can be hard going all the same.

Another confusion about testing is exactly what testing
you will be offered in your area. It's not a question I can
answer for you. Almost all women will now be offered routine
ultrasound scanning during pregnancy, but whilst some will
have just one scan, between 16 and 20 weeks, others will have
as many as three scans during their pregnancy. A good many
women over 37 will be offered amniocentesis, but some
hospitals have a policy of only offering amnios to women over
40, whilst others offer them to all women aged 35 and over.
Some areas undertake AFP testing as standard, others offer
triple test to all women, whilst others restrict triple test to older
women. One thing is for sure: you cannot insist on testing.
Testing is available privately, for instance triple test, through
the University of Leeds Down's Syndrome Screening Service
(see Appendix I), but remember to ask who you will be able to
talk to about the results of the test before you get in too deep.

> *'Because I was forty and so aware of the risks of
> Down's, I completely denied my pregnancy until after I'd
> had the amnio results.'*

Whether to test or not may be a relatively easy decision if
you have genetic disease in the family. If you are an older
mother, you may feel very ambivalent about testing. On the

one hand, you know that your risk of having a handicapped baby is increased. On the other hand, you may be acutely aware that if you do have a miscarriage as a result of testing, it may take you a long time to get pregnant again, if at all. If this is how you feel, you may prefer to have either nuchal fold screening by ultrasound at 10 weeks (details are given later), or alternatively triple test at 16 weeks. Both will give you some idea of your individual risk estimate (as opposed to the general one for your age), which may help you make a decision as to whether to live with your risk or go ahead with further testing.

Having reviewed some of the dilemmas, let's deal with the practicalities. Although you'll find information about each type of testing procedure, the emphasis is on the problems likely to be thrown up by each of them. Let's start with the one most pregnant women are likely to encounter – ultrasound.

Ultrasound Scanning

As I have indicated, almost all pregnant women will have an ultrasound scan at some time during their pregnancy. For many women, the first scan has become rather a celebratory event, a meet-your-baby-on-the-monitor session. When you are pregnant, especially for the first time, it is very difficult in those early months before you feel the baby moving to appreciate that there really is a baby in there. Seeing your baby on scan makes the connection with reality and it can be a very moving and exciting experience. But putting you in touch with your baby isn't what scanning is about. The scan operator is checking for signs of abnormality, just as much as for signs of good health.

First let's be clear about scanning in general, because there seems to be some confusion about what scans are for and what they can and can't tell you.

There are three levels of scanning and each can be carried out at any stage of pregnancy. The basic difference is not in the quality of machinery being used but in the skill of the operator, which is the single most important factor in scanning accuracy. What you are trying to do with an ultrasound scan is interpret a three-dimensional structure (your baby) from a two-dimensional image (what you and the operator see on the screen). There are any number of pitfalls for the unwary, and ultrasound diagnosis is much harder than you might imagine.

The most basic scanning is undertaken by midwives and GPs in non-hospital settings. Such a scan would probably take no more than five minutes or so and would merely establish that there was a baby in the womb and whether or not there was a fetal heart beat (you can see the heart pulsating on scan). Anybody can use scanning equipment – that bit is easy – but to interpret scans properly you need to be properly trained (i.e. something more than just an instruction course from the rep who sold the equipment). A friend of mine nearly had heart failure when the practice nurse, armed with a portable scanner, told her that she was expecting triplets. A visit to the local hospital quickly established that there was only one baby. You might think this a rather far-fetched story, but the combination of inexperience and a rapidly moving baby can cause all sorts of problems. Only the most severe of malformations could be seen using this type of scanning procedure. It is unlikely that the operators in these cases have sufficient skills to interpret what they see with any accuracy and this sort of scanning would not constitute a screen for physical malformation in your baby.

The next level of scanning (level 2 fetal anomaly scanning) would be carried out at a district general hospital. It would take on average about 15–20 minutes and would be done by someone specially trained in the use of ultrasound. The scan operator is more likely to be a technician than a doctor.

You will normally automatically be included for level 2 scanning in a DGH as part of your routine antenatal care package. You don't have to ask for it, even if you are just having GP care.

You may wonder whether level 2 anomaly scanning is enough, and whether level 3 scanning should be sought if you really want to be extra sure. The way it works is that level 2 scanning should trigger level 3 scanning if that is required. Unless you were particularly anxious, or had some family history that suggested level 3 scanning, you would not normally be offered this level of scan; nor is this level of scanning yours by right.

Level 3 scanning is of a very high quality and is offered at specialist centres only (usually teaching hospitals). The operator will be a doctor who has considerable experience of ultrasound and who will be able confidently to diagnose fetal abnormalities with a high degree of accuracy. This type of ultrasound is used in conjunction with CVS (see page 101) and with fetal treatments such as transfusion.

This makes it sound as though fetal anomaly scanning is all that ultrasound is used for. In reality, ultrasound has hundreds of uses, including assessing your baby's general wellbeing (for instance, following a threatened miscarriage), age and rate of growth, locating the placenta, etc. But remember, each scan has a specific purpose – if you are having a scan because you have been bleeding, your baby is not necessarily being checked for abnormality as well.

'Having to have a full bladder was agony.'

'How I didn't piddle all over their floor I'll never know.'

Scans in early pregnancy require a full bladder as this makes for a better picture. As these comments indicate, the only real problem with ultrasound is having an incredibly full bladder – and then having someone lean on it with an ultrasound transducer (that's the bit that they glide over your tummy). If you really are bursting, tell someone and ask if you can pee at least some of it away – but don't whatever you do let it all go, otherwise you'll be fed glasses of water until your bladder is full again. Ideally you should be wearing separates; that way you will only have to hitch up your top, and undo and lower your trousers or skirt a little. A dress has to be hitched up above your waist.

Most fetal anomaly scanning is undertaken between 16 and 20 weeks. People sometimes ask me why they can't get it over and done with much earlier in pregnancy. The answer is that if you scanned at 12 weeks, you wouldn't be able to see many of the body's structures in the required detail, whereas you can at, say, 20 weeks. The exceptions to this are some urinary tract and kidney problems which may not be apparent on scan until after 30 weeks.

'The first time we saw Charlie on the scan, we both cried. It was wonderful.'

For many of those in our survey, their first ultrasound scan was a magical experience. But ultrasound can throw up lots of difficulties too. Let's take the thoughtless remarks first. Sometimes doctors and scan operators are a bit less sensitive than they ought to be. They just think that they are being cheery. You, on the other hand, may take what they say as being gospel medical-speak and begin to panic when they say something like, 'Goodness, you've got a big one in here.' They think you will be pleased to know that you have a fine healthy baby. You, however, are beginning to think along the lines of impossible labours, 10 lb babies and the like. What you have to accept is that in general these remarks have no medical meaning; they're just chat. If they had medical meaning, they would be far more specific. And one more thing – although ultrasound can be used to measure babies, it is not a good predictor of final birthweight.

The next thing is, can you, can't you? – tell the sex of the baby, that is. Even the most skilled operators occasionally get it wrong. All those loops of umbilical cord between the legs can be very deceiving. Many units do not allow scan operators to tell parents the sex of their baby in case they get it wrong. Others will tell you if you ask; but remember, the only way to determine a baby's sex definitively is to undertake karyotyping.

After your scan the operator may tell you that it has not been possible to see what was required and you may be asked to come back for another one. Don't jump to the conclusion that something must be wrong with your baby. It's just that babies can be downright uncooperative and awkward sometimes, lying in positions which make it very difficult to get a good screen image. There's a similar problem if women are very overweight.

Scan operators work through a checklist when undertaking fetal anomaly scanning. People sometimes assume that looking at a scan picture is rather like looking at a baby through the glass of a goldfish bowl – you can see everything. In truth it's not like this and whilst, for instance, you can see the head in about 95 per cent of scans, you can only see a full four-chamber view of the heart (which is what you need to check whether it has formed properly) in less than half of scans. Thus there will be a gap on the operator's checklist, hence the need to call women back sometimes.

Women usually realise when something on scan is causing anxiety, partly because their own anxiety makes them particularly sensitive. There's a tendency, too, for professionals suddenly to scan in silence, which can be very unnerving, although they may simply be concentrating hard, to be absolutely sure of their findings. Couples may have had it explained, prior to the scan, that it will not be possible to tell them immediately what the scan shows. This does not mean that an abnormal finding is expected, merely that the scan operator is a technician rather than a doctor who may not have had the training required to interpret scan information. In this situation, parents will be asked to wait whilst the appropriate professional is found. Alternatively another appointment, usually within twenty-four hours, will be made.

'They said that the baby might have hydrocephalus [an excessive amount of fluid within the skull] but couldn't be sure. I had several scans over a period of a month. We were sick with worry. Finally, one day I had a scan and they said his head looked perfectly normal now. And that was that, we were expected to just forget all that worry. I wish I'd never had a scan in the first place.'

Waiting a day or so is agonising enough. An equally difficult situation is when a question mark is raised about your baby's health during a scan and you are asked to return, not immediately, but in a couple of weeks' time to 'see how things are getting on'. For example, the operator may say something like, 'This head is rather big', or 'This baby is rather small', and suggest an appointment in a fortnight for a further scan. You may be very alarmed and fear the worst. What you need to know is that babies don't grow in quite the same way as those nice smooth growth charts would suggest. They grow in fits and starts, and usually by the time of the next scan everything is back on track. Remember that growth charts are composite charts, not individual charts, and all the blips that you would find in a specific baby's growth chart have been ironed out by the mass statistics involved in compiling national growth charts.

Some parents say before they have a scan that they don't want to know about any problem which is marginal, and which the obstetrician thinks will resolve itself. This approach is very sound. An example here is something called a choroid plexus cyst, which shows up on scan as a little dark hole in the brain. If it is a small one, it will almost certainly resolve itself, although not usually until about 24 weeks by which time, of course, you would be completely witless. If it is larger, there is an association with certain chromosome abnormalities which would suggest the need for karyotyping, which would probably be carried out immediately. Some hospitals have a policy of not telling a woman if there is a choroid plexus cyst less than a certain size, simply because it will almost certainly resolve and to tell the woman would cause untold and unnecessary anxiety.

Can ultrasound scans be wrong? As I have said, with ultrasound scanning, it's not the image or the machinery that is a problem, it is the interpretation of that image. If something grave, or even something that just worries you, is found on a scan, you should ask to have a second scan by another consultant or to be referred to someone with specialist ultrasound skills. This is the moment to insist on level 3 scanning; but in practice you shouldn't have any difficulty in being referrred.

If you do have a problem diagnosed, such as poor fetal growth, you may find yourself having lots of scans. You may be alarmed by this, having read scare stories about ultrasound in the press. There was a finding that showed that 30 per cent more babies who had been scanned in the womb were left-handed than might be predicted by chance alone. This was meant to imply some degree of brain damage. Being left-handed myself, I have to say that I personally do not regard this as a sign of brain damage, although some might argue otherwise. Ultrasound probably is overused; it is probably being used as a substitute for routine skills in many settings, rather than as a very valuable addition to those skills. There's precious little evidence that routine use of ultrasound reduces perinatal mortality.

On the other hand, if you have a high risk pregnancy, ultrasound can mean the difference between having a baby and not having one. I think you have to be sensible about this. The evidence of harm from ultrasound is thin on the ground. Women have been having ultrasound scans for many years now in pregnancy, and there has been no increase in childhood cancers and the proportion of low birthweight babies has hardly changed, which makes a nonsense of some of ultrasound's opponents' wilder claims. Nevertheless, ultrasound is emphatically not just a tool for bonding with your baby and it should be treated with respect. Even if it were to be harmful in the long term, such risks are as nothing compared to the dangers that your baby faces right now if you have a high risk pregnancy, so if you are having to have lots of scans for some reason, dismiss worries about ultrasound from your mind completely.

Before leaving ultrasound, a word about three newer developments. The first is Doppler ultrasound. Although this works on the same principle as conventional ultrasound, noise is generated rather than image, and this noise is translated as a series of patterns on a monitor. Doppler is principally used to track the bloodflow to the baby through the placenta, and also bloodflow within the baby. Abnormal Doppler flow wave-forms are associated with growth retardation and with some specific abnormalities. However, all attempts to introduce Doppler as a mass screening technique have failed. None-theless, it has an extremely valuable role in high risk pregnancies and this is where you may meet Doppler for the first time.

Vaginal ultrasonography involves the use of a transducer which, instead of gliding over your tummy, is put in the vagina. Vaginal ultrasound is used in gynaecological work (to assess ovulation in those with fertility problems, for instance) and also in early pregnancy. It sounds unpleasant, but it isn't, so don't be alarmed if someone suggests it. The pictures are rather better than would be obtained by conventional ultrasound, and another advantage is that copious water drinking is not required, since a full bladder is not necessary for this type of scanning.

Finally, soft signs. As I indicated before, soft signs are small physical 'markers' which may point towards a particular condition, such as Down's Syndrome or other chromosome abnormality, even though chromosomes can't be 'seen' on ultrasound. The most interesting development in this field is called nuchal fold screening. Babies who have Down's Syndrome have a thickened fold of skin around the neck (the so-called nuchal fold), which appears as a dark bar round the neck from early pregnancy. At the time of writing, a major trial is in progress to assess whether nuchal fold screening at 10 weeks with ultrasound would be a more effective screening method than triple test. My money is on nuchal fold screening.

No soft sign, I know, but during my first pregnancy I was scanned by one of Britain's leading ultrasound experts. As he did the scan, he remarked on the baby's tongue. Sure enough, on the screen you could see this tongue in almost perpetual motion. My husband groaned, 'Not another one like her, please.' From the day that my son uttered his first word, he's never stopped talking. Curious that. Could he have got it from me? I doubt it.

Triple Test

'I got into a complete state over triple test. The results were very worrying, although everything was fine in the end.'

The test that seems to have caused our survey respondents more problems than any other is the triple test. Whilst some health messages pass us by, others are received loud and clear, lodging themselves irretrievably in the national psyche. One such is the fact that there is an increased likelihood of having a baby with a chromosome abnormality, such as Down's Syndrome, with increasing maternal age. The figures are dramatic. Roughly, they are a risk of 1 in 1,000 at 27, rising to 1 in 350 by the age of 35, 1 in 100 at 40 and 1 in 25 at 45. You'd think, given these figures, that most Down's babies would be born to older women. Actually over 60 per cent of Down's babies are born to women under 35. Whilst older women should be aware of an increased risk, it is a risk that is overplayed. Part of the problem is that in devising a risk figure, all women of a particular age are lumped together in a convenient medical pigeonhole that says 'These women are all aged 40, therefore their risk is X'. In truth, all women of 40 are not the same. They have differing risks. Triple test is a way of arriving at an individual estimate of risk. In doing so, some 70 per cent of women aged 40 are shown to have a risk rate lower than a woman of 35. Triple test can of course also be used to give an individual risk estimate to younger women. Thus women who have previously never considered themselves at risk may find themselves suddenly in a high risk bracket, and women who thought that they had a very high risk may find that the converse is true. Women treat risk estimates in different ways: if you are 25, a risk of 1 in 400 may seem very high to you, whilst if you are 40 it will seem low. But risk and actuality are two different things and the important thing to remember about triple test (or indeed any other screening test) is that being 'at increased risk' does not mean that you are carrying a handicapped baby. Only a direct diagnostic test, such as karyotyping following amniocentesis, can tell you that for sure. On the other hand, being deemed 'low risk' is not a guarantee that your baby is healthy. Confused? An awful lot of you were.

Triple test, also known as the Barts test (because it was initially devised at Bart's Hospital), involves the measurement of three separate blood chemicals (alphafetoprotein (AFP), unconjugated oestriol (uE3) and human chorionic gonado-trophin (hCG)) in a sample of the mother's blood. The blood test can be carried out at any time between 15 and 23 weeks, but is most often undertaken at about 16 weeks. Accurate dating of your pregnancy is essential because, in order to arrive at your individual risk ratio for Down's Syndrome, the levels of all three chemicals in your blood, plus your exact gestation, plus your age, are fed into a computer for calculation. If your dates are wrong it can affect the validity of the result. Other situations where triple test results need special interpretation are if you are carrying twins, if you are diabetic, and whether you have had a previous baby with either Down's or a neural tube defect. For technical reasons, triple test cannot be interpreted properly if you have had an amniocentesis during this pregnancy. Maternal weight and ethnic origin both influence the result, but adjustments are made for these factors when the test is interpreted.

The level of AFP alone is used to determine whether there is an increased risk of NTD, thereby detecting almost all cases of anencephaly and four out of five cases of spina bifida.

Printed results are given to all women undertaking triple test within about ten days. The results are shown as either screen negative or screen positive. The important thing to understand *before* you have triple test is that a screen positive result does not mean that you are carrying a handicapped baby – it simply means that further testing is advised. About 1 in 20 of all women screened will have a screen positive result due to an increased risk of Down's Syndrome. The vast majority of these women do not have an affected pregnancy. On average, only 1 in 70 women with a screen positive result will have a Down's affected pregnancy. Three out of every five Down's pregnancies will be detected, but two out of three will not. If this doesn't sound like a very high detection rate to you, remember that screening by triple test detects twice as many Down's affected pregnancies as does screening on the basis of a woman's age alone. Detection rates also increase with age.

A test result is screen negative if the AFP level is not high, and therefore an NTD is not suspected, or if the risk of Down's Syndrome is less than 1 in 250. But 1 in 1,700 of women who screen negative will in fact have a baby with Down's. As I have already explained, only four out of five cases of spina bifida will be detected.

Just a cautionary note about numbers. You will be given an exact risk ratio. A risk less than 1 in 250 means (conversely for non-mathematicians like me) a bigger number, like 1 in 400, or 1 in 5,000 or 1 in 10,000. A risk greater than 1 in 250, that is, a positive result, is a smaller number, like 1 in 100 or 1 in 50. Let's be clear too about what 1 in 50 means. It means that 49 women will have healthy babies.

So what do you do if you screen positive? It depends somewhat on your perspective. If you are 45, with a screen positive result but a risk ratio of 1 in 100, you may decide to do nothing further, given that your individual risk odds are a good deal better than the age-specific odds of 1 in 25. If however, at 45, you decide that you do want a bit more investigation, but not any sort of invasive testing, you could ask to have a detailed ultrasound scan, looking for Down's Syndrome soft signs. Again, you will not get a conclusive answer, but you might be sufficiently reassured to forego an amnio, or alternatively decide that there is so much doubt that only a definitive diagnosis will do, and go on to an amnio.

On the other hand, if you are 25, a risk of 1 in 100 may seem massive and you may want diagnostic testing. And here's the rub. If you have an amniocentesis, the results will take three weeks to come through. So, if you got your triple test results at, say, 18 weeks, your amnio result won't arrive until you are 21 weeks. I personally think that a three-week wait for results under these circumstances is torture of the worst sort. Your sanity may, however, be slightly restored by immediate detailed ultrasound scanning which may at least reassure you that the odds of the amnio result being negative are very high. Under these circumstances, you would need to have the scan in a tertiary referral centre, where an obstetrician specialising in fetal medicine is located. (The Royal College of Obstetricians and Gynaecologists – see Appendix I – maintains a list of these.) The other possible route is to have cordocentesis (which you'll find fully explained later in this chapter), because the results can be available in two days. Cordocentesis is only possible after 18 weeks, and once again you would only find the expertise necessary to undertake it in a large teaching hospital. Ask your obstetrician to refer you – they are normally very sympathetic to this sort of request, but expect to have to travel.

Triple test is causing enormous problems at the moment, mostly I think because it is not being adequately explained in advance. Prior to triple test, amnios were being offered to about 5 per cent of women (based on age alone). The general plot is that once triple test is fully introduced, the same percentage, i.e. 5 per cent, of women will have amnios, but they will be women at higher risk rather than just older women. That's the theory. What's happening in practice is that women with a screen positive result are unwilling (and can you blame them) to wait for the results of amnios and are besieging tertiary referral centres in an effort to get a quicker fix on their baby's health, either via detailed ultrasound scanning or by cordocentesis. Thus there is a greater demand for diagnostic testing than, I suspect, anyone ever envisaged. We shall see.

MSAFP

Whilst we are on the subject of triple test, it is worth tackling the other maternal blood test, maternal serum AFP (MSAFP). This is the screening test for neural tube defects, the family of handicaps that includes anencephaly (a lethal condition in which the cover of the baby's brain fails to form properly) and spina bifida. AFP is a protein which is made by the baby's liver and excreted with the baby's urine into the pool of amniotic fluid. There are large quantities of AFP in the skin and muscles of babies and if there is an open hole in the skin, as there is with most NTDs, it leaks out so that much larger concentrations than normal are found in the fluid. Some of this AFP crosses the mother's placenta into her bloodstream. The higher the concentration of AFP in the amniotic fluid, the higher the level of AFP likely to be found in the mother's blood.

AFP testing is usually undertaken between 16 and 18 weeks. Some districts have chosen to replace AFP testing with triple test (which simply involves the measurement of two further chemicals from the same single blood sample). However, AFP screening has never been a universal test simply because its incidence varies so greatly across the country, from just 2 per 1,000 in London to 7–8 per 1,000 in parts of Wales. The reason for this geographical variation is not fully understood, although one thing is for sure: there is no single cause for these handicaps, which arise through a complex interaction of inherited and environmental factors.

One of the problems of AFP testing is the way the results are dispensed. Unlike triple test, there is no 'bit of paper' which gives you a result. Rather unsatisfactorily it is a 'don't call us, we'll call you' situation; that is, assume that everything is fine unless you hear otherwise. This sort of approach can leave you feeling anxious and concerned for weeks. It may be possible for you to leave a stamped addressed card with someone which can be sent to you on receipt of a negative result.

AFP results are expressed as a number that gives a risk rate, usually as something called an MoM or Multiple of the Median. This sounds much more complicated than it is – a way of expressing your risk relative to others. This MoM number can be adjusted according to your weight, race, age and week of pregnancy.

As to the results themselves, here come the problems. The first thing you need to know is that, just like triple test, a positive result does not mean that you are carrying a handicapped baby. In fact, nine out of ten women who have a raised level of AFP do not have a handicapped baby.

Unfortunately AFP testing isn't very specific and there is quite an overlap between normal babies and babies with an NTD.

Let's look at some of the reasons why you might have an elevated AFP level. One of the most common is that women are more advanced in pregnancy than they thought they were. AFP levels rise in a set and predictable way with gestation, and if you think you are 16 weeks, but are actually 18 weeks, your AFP level will seem very high for 16 weeks, but be quite normal for 18 weeks. Another good reason for higher than normal AFP levels is that there is more than one baby. Also, previous bleeding in the pregnancy, perhaps a threatened miscarriage, also seems to produce elevated AFP readings. Very rarely − and I mean very rarely − where high AFP levels are found in conjunction with other signs, such as a very small amount of amniotic fluid, the baby may have a more serious health problem and this would need further investigation. However, having said all of this, you should be aware that, at birth, no reason at all can be found for elevated AFP levels in 50 per cent of babies whose mothers' blood contained high AFP levels in pregnancy. Does this mean that, if no cause can be found for elevated AFP, you should ignore the result? Evidence suggests that the finding should be viewed in rather the same way as you view a hazard road sign, like the one with the leaping deer on it. It doesn't mean that the deer is waiting to jump in front of your car around the next corner; just that you should be aware of the possibility. In the same way, high AFP levels are sometimes indicators of hazards ahead. For instance, it is strongly suspected that problems with the placenta are responsible for some unexplained high AFP levels. Many obstetricians would therefore think it prudent to monitor your pregnancy, and particularly the baby's growth, more carefully following such a finding.

What if you have a very low AFP result? Low AFP levels

are associated with Down's Syndrome, but the very reason that triple test includes two other chemicals as well as AFP is because AFP is such a poor predictive test on its own of Down's, with an unacceptable number of false positives.

> 'I had a nightmare time with the AFP test. The level was very low and I was told it could be a Down's baby. I never knew anything about dates being so important, and it was only after I'd gone into a blind panic and they'd done a scan, that everyone realised my dates were wrong. My baby was fine but I never stopped worrying the whole pregnancy.'

If you do have an abnormal AFP result, what next? Firstly remember, if you possibly can, that nine out of ten women with high AFP levels have normal babies and that what you are about to go through is the only route to the reassurance you seek. One of the first steps might be a scan to check your dates, and then a retest. A repeat test for a high level will either produce a result within normal limits if your dates were incorrect, or continue to be high. If the problem was a low AFP, retesting is not an option, because AFP levels rise as your pregnancy progresses anyway. In the past, amniocentesis used to be the next step because, as I indicated earlier, AFP levels are much higher and less subject to error in amniotic fluid, which is why a sample of amniotic fluid was required. Results may take as much as three weeks if karyotyping is involved, but be available much more quickly if all that is required is a simple measure of AFP in the fluid. Nowadays, however, if an NTD is suspected, first stop would be a detailed ultrasound scan. Anancephaly should be spotted instantly; spina bifida is rather more difficult. This is because there are both open and closed lesions, and the latter in particular is not easy to spot on scan. A high level of ultrasound scanning expertise is required for a scan of this sort, so you might be referred to a hospital specialising in Fetal Medicine.

With anencephaly, the prognosis is not in doubt. Anencephalic babies die either at birth or within a couple of hours of birth. But with spina bifida, decisions are far more difficult because it is usually not possible to diagnose the extent of handicap prior to birth. Down's Syndrome is another handicap with a variable prognosis. Although some work is being undertaken at present relating extensive study of fetal movements to severity of subsequent handicap, very few doctors, if any, would be able to tell you with any certainty how severe your child's handicap is likely to be.

The final sorts of testing are the invasive procedures – amniocentesis, cordocentesis and chorionic villus sampling (CVS). These procedures all do the same thing; they are means of obtaining samples of the baby's tissue for further testing, either for karyotyping, for specific genetic testing, or for testing for metabolic disease. Fewer than 10 per cent of women will experience these types of testing, so the account of them in this book is necessarily rather brief. Each procedure is, however, dealt with in much more detail in my previous book *The Antenatal Testing Handbook* (Pan, 1993). Mostly when people ask me about testing, they ask about the risks of these particular procedures.

Cordocentesis

Let's deal with cordocentesis first, as this is by no means routine. If you've got to the stage of having cordocentesis you are already well down the testing trail. Cordocentesis involves taking a sample of the baby's blood, under ultrasound guidance, from the umbilical vein. Because the baby's blood vessels are so fragile and so tiny, this can't be undertaken before 18 weeks. Reasons for having cordocentesis are usually that you have already had an adverse test result, for instance a positive triple test result, or some suspicious soft signs on ultrasound, and fast karyotyping is required. Between 1 and 2 women in every 100 having the procedure will have a spontaneous miscarriage.

CVS

Chorionic villus sampling (CVS) involves taking a small piece of placental tissue (the placenta should be the same tissue-type as the baby), either in a procedure very similar to an amnio or, and this is less common in Britain, through the vagina. This is called transcervical CVS. There isn't a great deal of difference in terms of safety between the two techniques, providing, that is, that it is the operator's preferred technique. Basically, it boils down to 'practice makes perfect', and if the person under-taking your CVS has done nothing but transcervical CVS, believe me, that immediately makes transcervical the safer technique *in his hands*.

CVS is carried out from 9 weeks of pregnancy up to 13 weeks for transabdominal CVS, and up to 11 weeks of transcervical. There has been some concern recently over limb defects in babies born to women who have had CVS in early pregnancy. The numbers involved are very small indeed and there seems to be a link between very early CVS and these problems. As a result, CVS is usually not undertaken before 10 weeks.

Because CVS is undertaken in the first trimester, when

miscarriage rates are at their peak, it has always been difficult to assess whether miscarriage is the result of the procedure or a miscarriage that would have occurred anyway. The procedure loss rate is between 2 and 3 in every 100. Some very experienced centres would claim that their loss rate was lower. As I hinted earlier, operator skill is all and you should certainly ensure that you have CVS undertaken in a centre with an extensive experience of the technique.

Because CVS involves taking living placental tissue, and therefore no culturing is required, in theory results could be available in a couple of days. However, results take a week in most cases, and up to three weeks in some. This is because there was some concern over result accuracy in the early days of CVS and rigorous checking and double-checking are undertaken.

A normal CVS result means that there are the normal number of chromosomes and that they are of the normal shape and size. No information about specific single gene defects will have been obtained unless this was the reason for the CVS in the first place. No information about the presence or absence of physical abnormality will have been obtained.

Amniocentesis

Finally to amniocentesis. Of all the invasive procedures, this is the most familiar. During pregnancy a baby luxuriates in its own private pond. The pond is enclosed within a sac made of amnion which is stretchy, waterproof and very strong. At the beginning of pregnancy it is the cells that line the amniotic sac which make the fluid, but at about 12 weeks the baby takes over, gulping the fluid down and then passing it, making a little more along the way as it does so. Thus amniotic fluid consists pretty much of baby's recycled urine. Because the baby is constantly wriggling about, cells get rubbed off its skin – in the same way that our skin cells rub off when we're washing ourselves in the bath – and these living cells then float about in the amniotic fluid. If you took a sample of your bath water you'd be almost certain to find some of your cells in it; the same is true of the baby's cells and amniotic fluid. Amniocentesis is a very familiar and fairly straightforward procedure and is carried out at about 16 weeks, or any stage thereafter. Earlier amniocenteses are available in some teaching hospitals from about 10 weeks. As yet, these are still the subject of trial and there has been some concern as to whether taking fluid at such an early stage of pregnancy will result in an increased rate of respiratory disease at birth. So far this hasn't been the case, but the procedure is still relatively uncommon at such an early gestation.

The problem about amniocentesis is that these cells have to be cultured, and the culturing process takes at least two weeks, meaning a delay of at least three weeks between test and result. It is the delay that those who responded to our survey found so distressing. Should the result be positive, and if you decide on a termination you will be close to 20 weeks pregnant and will have to go through an induced labour which is a grim experience.

'I never knew three weeks could feel like three years.'

Amniocentesis is the safest of all the invasive procedures with a risk of spontaneous miscarriage of less than 1 in 100 in the best hands. Despite everyone's best efforts, about 1 in 100 cell samples will fail to culture at all. Although a further amniocentesis might be offered, most women would probably rather not go through it all again at such a late stage of pregnancy. There are several possibilities, some of which are dependent on your reason for having an amniocentesis in the first place. If it was for maternal age alone, you might prefer to have a very detailed ultrasound scan at this stage. This is, as I have explained, a screening procedure only and can only reassure you rather than be completely definite about the presence or absence of chromosome disorders such as Down's. If you want definitive diagnosis, karyoptying is the only sure way, which would mean either a further amnio or possibly, if you felt that time was very much against you, cordocentesis (see page 100), which is available only in centres specialising in fetal medicine (a list of these is available from the Royal College of Obstetricians and Gynaecologists – see Appendix I). Another rather similar, but more unusual problem (occurring in 1 in 600 procedures), which demand much the same approach, is maternal cell contamination of the sample – i.e. some of your cells got into the sample.

As I have said, amniocentesis is probably the safest invasive procedure. Normally, the little hole in the amniotic sac made by the needle closes up by itself, very quickly. Sometimes it doesn't and amniotic fluid may continue to leak out via the little hole, albeit at a very slow rate. This is not unusual in the first few hours after an amnio, but if the leak continues, tell someone straightaway. It doesn't mean that something awful is going to happen, but it does need to be watched closely. Very occasionally women continue to leak tiny amounts of fluid throughout the pregnancy thereafter, with the baby being perfectly fine. Amnionitis – an infection in the amniotic fluid – occurs in only 1 in 1,000 cases. If you have a raised temperature following an amnio, report it, just in case.

For some women, who have had some of the testing procedures outlined above, termination will be an option. It is a miserable, distressing experience although hospital staff do all they can to make it less so. I have outlined the details of the termination procedure in my book *The Antenatal Testing Handbook*. Alternatively, you might like to contact SATFA (Support around Termination for Abnormality – see Appendix I). Although you might feel that a decision needs to be taken quickly, it is important that you take your time, and a week or even a bit longer will make no difference.

You can, if you want, see testing as a form of reassurance; but it is definitely reassurance bought at a price, and that price is the increased anxiety and concern that waiting for results inevitably brings. Treat testing with respect.

6

Common Pregnancy Problems

You will note immediately that I have titled this section 'common pregnancy problems' rather than 'minor pregnancy problems'. The sort of problems with which this chapter is concerned are those which, truth to speak, are not life-threatening for either mother or baby, but which nevertheless do not deserve the epithet 'minor' since, as far as I am concerned, they probably collectively cause more distress amongst pregnant women than most 'major' problems put together.

The psychology of these problems is interesting. Because they affect you and not your baby, sympathy and concern seem to be dished out in extremely limited measure by those around you. There's no two ways about it – pregnancy can be a bitch. The only cure for most of the following conditions is not to be pregnant. But you know this, and there's no turning back now. Here then is some practical help for the miserable moments in your pregnancy.

Cramp

Cramp is a painful spasm in a muscle caused by excessive and prolonged contraction of the muscle fibres. It is experienced by almost half of pregnant women at some time in their pregnancy. It seems to strike when you are in bed at night, often when you are asleep and especially when you point your toes. The pain is excruciating, sudden and, as you leap from the bed with a banshee shriek, a cause of considerable alarm to your partner. These cramps may recur repeatedly for days or even a few weeks, but the good news is that they will almost invariably disappear as suddenly as they appeared.

Theories as to their cause are numerous, with mineral deficiency being almost universally cited as the prime culprit. Let's be practical about this, however. Can half of all pregnant women be mineral deficient? And why do cramps come and then suddenly go, without any obvious change of diet? Why are some women affected at one stage of pregnancy and others at another? The deficiency story simply doesn't hold water. Nevertheless, calcium or calcium salt tablets are frequently dispensed as a cure. Certainly calcium is essential to muscle function, but treatment with calcium tablets has never been proved to work. Salt (sodium chloride) tablets were found in one study to be more effective than a placebo but these results have not been confirmed.

The following self-help measures may be useful. To prevent cramps, try rolling your foot over a tennis ball or milk bottle several times as you watch TV in the evening. Try some leg stretching exercises too. When cramp strikes, sit on the floor with your legs out in front of you and pull your toes towards you. Pulling the muscles in the opposite way like this should get rid of the immediate pain. Then sit with your knees up and rub your leg gently – don't be tempted to rub too hard. This is one of the few pregnancy problems where your partner can provide practical help, so accept it gratefully.

Restless Legs

I wrote about restless legs once in a magazine; one small paragraph attracted more letters than almost any other piece I've ever written, so I know how big a problem it is, especially in pregnancy. Basically your legs won't relax, they feel as if they have to be on the move, and the only relief is getting up and walking around. Sitting for long periods seems to trigger the discomfort which is often worst at night. There is no single cure and I can't offer you any science, either as to cause or resolution. Some people benefit from warming their legs, others from cooling them, but the important point to make is that you are perfectly normal, you are not about to fall to pieces, and it will go away.

Faintness

Some women are prone to fainting, others are not. Pregnancy makes you particularly vulnerable to fainting, partly because of altered blood circulation but also because of the size and weight of the pregnancy pressing on the blood return to the heart. If you are a non-fainting type, this may be a new and very alarming experience which you feel must indicate some serious underlying disorder. Not so.

There are a number of situations which have the potential to make anyone feel faint, never mind when you are carrying a ten-ton baby inside you as well. These include standing for long periods, being stuck in overcrowded hot places and being in smoky atmospheres. Recognise such risk situations in advance. You may not be able to avoid them, but try and locate a chair and sit down for a bit if you can, or get out for some fresh air. Although it sounds completely daft, breathing in and out of a paper bag works brilliantly. The science behind it is that faintness often follows a period of hyperventilation (breathing more quickly than normal). Rapid breathing removes too much carbon dioxide from the body. Breathing in and out of a paper bag means that you are forcing yourself to breathe your expired air, which is largely carbon dioxide, which rapidly restores your carbon dioxide balance and moderates your breathing. Lying down with your feet higher than your heart is also a rapid route to recovery, but not always practical. Putting your head down between your legs when sitting is also effective. After fainting, drink something containing sugar such as a fizzy drink or sweet tea.

You may have been able to miss meals with impunity before you got pregnant, but when pregnant long gaps between meals and the consequent fall in blood sugar are another cause of fainting. It's not often you'll have a genuine excuse for snacks between meals, so go for it. In addition, when you lie down the weight of the baby presses down on the blood returning to the heart, and if you get up suddenly the room may spin. Be aware that you need to be a bit slower when changing posture when pregnant.

Numbness and Tingling in the Hands

Numbness, tingling and weakness of the fingers is common in pregnancy. There are two causes; carpal tunnel syndrome affects the thumb, index and middle fingers and results from pressure on a nerve where it passes into the hand via a gap (the carpal tunnel) under a ligament in the wrist. The pressure is usually the result of fluid retention (oedema), but it may even be something as silly as wearing a narrow bra strap which bites into your shoulder, putting pressure on the nerve that serves the hand and fingers. Numbness and tingling, which is worse at night and first thing in the morning, can also be the result of traction on the nerve connections in the shoulder caused by the natural drooping of the shoulders in pregnancy. Physiotherapy and massage can be very helpful in relieving discomfort caused by both these conditions. Don't be backwards about coming forward – if you are having a lot of pain or if the tingling is affecting your daily life (you keep dropping things, etc.), ask to be referred for physiotherapy. Both conditions resolve spontaneously after delivery, although residual tingling may take a couple of weeks to disappear completely.

Blocked Nose

The increased levels of the hormone oestrogen mean that all the body's membranes, including those in the nose, become softer and thicker in pregnancy. This may lead to extra mucus in the nose and a blocked-up feeling. Try not to use decongestants because they tend to have a rebound effect, making the problem worse with repeated use. The best solution is to plonk yourself under a towel, over a bowl of boiling water, and inhale steam for ten minutes or so each day; add some eucalyptus oil if you like the smell.

Aches and Pains

Because pregnancy is a natural event, we assume that the body just gets on and copes with it. It's only when you are not feeling your best and your mother-in-law says something like,

'It's not surprising with that great thing pushing your insides about,' that you suddenly realise that yes, she is right. Your growing womb is enforcing all sorts of rigours on your body, some of which will probably cause you discomfort. However, in the general way of things, we dismiss our mother-in-law's wisdom as that of an ignoramus and immediately assume when we get discomfort that something must be wrong. A good many aches and pains in pregnancy are unfortunately part of reproductive life's rich tapestry. If pain is accompanied by bleeding, if pain is severe and continuous, or if pain starts suddenly, is sharp and is felt much more on one side of the abdomen than the other, seek help. Niggling pain is, however, much more likely to be pregnancy induced than pregnancy threatening.

Your womb is suspended from the abdominal wall by ligaments. When these are stretched or perhaps strained during early pregnancy you may experience quite sharp pain, especially when you turn suddenly. If this is persistent, get your GP to check it, just to reassure yourself that there isn't another cause. Avoiding sudden jerky movements, drawing your knees up before turning over in bed, and trying to avoid walking downstairs with a heavy load will help. If the pain is persistent, the hospital may be able to provide an elastic support belt. This is called round ligament pain.

Joint pain is very common in pregnancy. The joints of the pelvis take a particular hammering, not only because of the unaccustomed weight (bodyweight is transmitted through them) but because changes in posture put additional strains upon them. Add to that the fact that these normally rigid joints become more lax in pregnancy because of the softening effect of pregnancy hormones, and you have a sure-fire recipe for back and joint pain. The three joints that cause particular problems are the pubic symphysis (just below your hairline at the front) and the two sacroiliac joints (in your lower back where the pelvis articulates with the sacrum).

Prevention is the key. Watch your posture; roll over in bed before standing up, rather than sitting bolt upright and then turning to stand. Build up those back muscles by swimming (but do crawl or backstroke; if you stick your neck out whilst doing breaststroke, you'll make things worse), and start the day by doing some pelvic tilt exercises (arch the spine, cat-like, whilst on all fours). Help yourself by realising your limitations. Don't carry heavy shopping (or if you do, use two bags not one); try and get someone else to lift your toddler out of the bath, or if you have to do it, really think about the lift, bending your knees and using your legs to minimise the strain on your back. Let someone else lift heavy things for you. There is something mesmerising about heavily pregnant women as far as men are concerned – particularly young men. They still believe all that Hollywood stuff about women going into labour at the drop of a hat (complete with groans and much clutching of stomach). If ever a man stands by while you struggle, go for the Oscar – just a bit of clutching will do. It works brilliantly. The point is, however, a serious one: strain a ligament and it'll take a surprisingly long time to heal. This is avoidable pain, so don't be proud; use one and all to avoid it.

Finally on the subject of back and joint pain, if you are doing something and you start to hurt – stop it. Your body is sending you the clearest possible warning signals and if you just grit your teeth and carry on it will be at your peril. The trouble is that life doesn't stop when you are pregnant; women want to be seen to be as competent as men, but when we are pregnant we are not superbeings, but vulnerable beings who find it a struggle to cope with job, family, household and life. This does not stop us claiming to be able to cope just fine. You don't get Brownie points for invincibility. Hoovering the stairs? Leave them. Taking all the shopping to the car in one trip? Make three trips and be late for your next appointment. Stripping the beds? Let the old man do it. It takes self-discipline to do this, but it really is worth it.

If your muscles were particularly lax before you got pregnant, if you are having twins or more, or just having a big baby, and if you also lead a very active life, consider using a maternity girdle (available from Mothercare). They're not fashionable, not pretty, but who cares. They can be very effective, particularly if you put them on at the start of the day, rather than just when the going gets tough.

The other source of pain comes from the activities of your baby. Breech babies, who sit upright in the womb, can be particularly awkward during pregnancy, kicking out in all directions. Babies who are in the right position, with their heads tucked down, loiter with intent to damage your ribcage until the very end of pregnancy, when, because the head drops down in the pelvis (engages), you can at last feel a little more comfortable. Earlier in pregnancy the bladder is often the butt of repeated assault. There are all sorts of jokes about giving birth to footballers (the whole Spurs team indeed) so active is this kicking, but actually it's no fun. You do get bruised and it can really hurt. The homeopathic remedy arnica is particularly good for this type of bruising. As for the kicking, there's not a lot you can do. Bless 'em!

Other Causes of Abdominal Pain

OVARIAN CYSTS

It is not uncommon for pregnant women to be told at their booking visit that they have an ovarian cyst. Apart from feeling that you have suddenly acquired three left feet, you may worry about the implications. Most ovarian cysts discovered at this stage of pregnancy are what might be termed leftovers. When the follicle releases an egg, it turns itself into a corpus luteum (yellow body) whose job it is to secrete progesterone, so maintaining the early pregnancy. After a while the placenta takes over this function, so that the corpus luteum becomes redundant. However, puffed up with the importance of its task, it may remain quite large. As pregnancy advances, the so-called luteal cyst disappears spontaneously. Only 10 per cent at most of ovarian cysts in pregnancy will require further investigation, and I have included ovarian cysts in this section because occasionally they can be a source of pain in early pregnancy (between the 8th and 16th week). Often ovarian cysts are attached to the ovary via little stalks. If these become twisted (torsion), the cysts lose their blood supply, causing sudden severe abdominal pain, which may sometimes radiate down the thigh. The pain usually diminishes after about twenty-four hours, but investigation via a laparoscope is indicated. The plot is usually to remove the cyst. Generally such surgery is carried out at about 14–16 weeks. The pregnancy is not normally affected.

FIBROIDS

Fibroids are found in association with about 5 per cent of pregnancies, the incidence being highest in Afro-Caribbean women over 35. These fibroids are often discovered during early scans and in general cause no further problem. They do enlarge and soften as the pregnancy increases, and if growth is particularly rapid, rather like the ovarian cyst story, their blood supply may become a bit precarious. The fibroid may then degenerate (usually in the second half of pregnancy) causing pain and a low grade fever. Bed rest, analgesia and abdominal ice packs are the usual treatment and the condition should resolve itself over a period of a week or so. This is called red degeneration and it is the reason why your fibroid(s) will be monitored closely during pregnancy if you have them. It is an unusual thing to happen, but once you know about it, it's not half as awful as you had imagined.

Heartburn

Over 70 per cent of pregnant women suffer from heartburn – or reflux oesophagitis, to give it its proper name. Pregnancy hormones make the ring of muscle that normally shuts the stomach off from the oesophagus more relaxed, allowing the acid contents of the stomach to escape into the lower oesophagus, resulting in the familiar burning pain. Heartburn is usually worse in the latter half of pregnancy, particularly when lying down or bending over. Late in pregnancy, the weight of the baby pressing on the digestive organs may in itself also cause heartburn. Luckily there are lots of self-help measures. Large heavy meals, particularly of very fatty or spiced foods, are bound to cause it, especially if eaten late at night, so try smaller, more frequent snacks instead, avoiding foods that seem to trigger bad attacks (peanut butter in my case, but it's different for everyone). Substituting a herbal tea, like fennel or peppermint, for tea or coffee after a meal can be very helpful. If you have to do a task that involves a lot of bending over, do it before a meal rather than immediately after. Heartburn is often most troublesome at night. Raising the head of the bed can be very effective – try putting a telephone directory under each of the top bedposts, or propping yourself up with pillows.

By all means take antacids, such as Rennies or Settlers, if it gets too much. They are not harmful to the baby, but paradoxically the more alkaline antacid you shovel in, the more acid your stomach produces in order to compensate, so don't rely on them too much. Having said that, the best time to take an antacid is about two to three hours after a meal and as you go to bed. Liquid antacids may be more effective and your GP will advise you which one to take. Curiously, if alkaline antacids prove completely ineffective, it is possible that your heartburn may be of the type caused by an excess of alkali in your stomach, in which case an acid remedy like cider vinegar may work.

This is a more unusual symptom of reflux oesophagitis, called 'water brash', in which you suddenly get a mouthful of clear, salty tasting fluid, which may make you feel rather sick. Using the same self-help measures as for heartburn should help avoid it.

Thrush

Thrush is caused by a yeast, candida albicans, and as you'll know if you are a bread maker, to get a yeast going you need to provide warmth and sugar. Unfortunately pregnancy provides both of these in abundance and thrush can become a real nuisance. Once established it is difficult to get rid of, so let's concentrate on prevention first.

One of the most important preventive measures is to wipe from front to back after using the loo as the bowel is a natural home for the thrush organism. Wash twice a day with cool water, avoiding soap, and be careful to wash after lovemaking. Make sure you dry yourself properly; it sounds mad, but a hairdryer on the cool setting is a good ploy. Use an anti-fungal cream like Canesten, available from your chemist without prescription, about twice a month to try and prevent attacks. Avoid bubble baths, scented talcs, etc. and also tight-fitting knickers or tights. It is always claimed that cotton underwear is best since it is supposed to absorb moisture and be cooler. But since when did Kim Basinger get her man on screen wearing voluminous cotton knickers? If it's a choice between thrush and clinging to the last vestiges of take-me-now womanhood, my advice is simple. Ditch the exotic lingerie during pregnancy, saving it for about six weeks after delivery, when anything that makes you feel even faintly erotic in your milk-leaking, washed–out–dishcloth state is to be commended.

If you get full-blown thrush, which is dreadfully itchy, try applying plain live yoghurt straight from the fridge on the affected areas. This won't cure the problem, but it will reduce the itching. Don't let thrush get out of hand, as it can get very sore and make you miserable. A short course of clotrimazole (Canestan) pessaries is very effective. Nystatin (Nystan) pessaries are slightly less effective but both are safe to use in pregnancy. Use the pessaries in conjunction with cream, and also treat your partner with cream in case he is re-infecting you. Oral thrush treatments (e.g. Diflucan, Sporanox) are highly effective but should not be used in pregnancy because of question marks over their possible effects on the baby. I should add that these concerns arise from animal studies and not hard and fast data on humans.

Varicose Veins

During pregnancy the blood vessels dilate and the walls bulge causing the bloodflow to become sluggish. Varicose veins may appear for the first time in pregnancy, either in the legs or the vulva, and either ache or itch or both. They may be apparent as bulging, bluish veins, or sometimes may not be particularly noticeable. They are perhaps the least attractive of these so-called 'minor problems', partly because, although they may regress after pregnancy, you know that they are never going to go away entirely. You put up with those discomforts which are part and parcel of pregnancy because that is what it takes, but being left with varicose veins seems grossly unfair. For many of us, it is also the all too obvious reminder of what is in store for us as we grow older. I developed a splendid varicose vein on my leg during pregnancy which my younger son points to and says, with some pride, 'I did that'; and so he did, the blighter (and the stretch marks for that matter).

Unfortunately varicose veins tend to run in families, so to some extent if that is what your genes say, you are stuck with it. However, there are things which you can do which will help. Sitting cross-legged won't cause varicose veins (contrary to popular belief), but if you have a tendency to them, it won't improve matters. Avoid wearing tight-fitting socks, or pop socks. When you sit down, always put your feet up, if possible, higher than your head. If you don't suffer from heartburn (as this remedy would exacerbate heartburn) raise the foot end of your bed, so that blood drains more easily back to the heart when you are lying down. Try not to stand for long periods, and do make sure that you have a good brisk walk every day as walking forces blood to return to the heart.

If you have varicose veins before you get pregnant, it would be a good idea to wear support tights during your pregnancy. The general idea with these is that you put them on whilst still in bed, rather than after you've got up, thus allowing the veins to drain first.

Varicose veins of the vulva are rotten and are one of those really unmentionable pregnancy problems which, outside a medical setting, you will find it difficult to share with anyone but your partner. They may be really painful, or make you feel that everything is about to fall out, or both. Lying down will relieve the pressure on them, but this isn't always possible. Ice packs may help (use a 1 lb pack of frozen petits pois), but one of the best remedies is to soak several soft sanitary towels with witch hazel, and put them in the fridge in a sealed plastic bag, for use as you need them. Despite their alarming appearance, these veins won't interfere with delivery, but the best news is that vulval varicose veins disappear completely soon after childbirth.

Piles

Piles are varicose veins of the rectum or anus. Once again they are a pretty unmentionable problem, causing itching, soreness and sometimes bleeding. Constipation really exacerbates the problem, so try and avoid getting constipated (see below). Apply a pile cream to the anus before passing a stool and clean the area afterwards by washing (bidets were invented for pregnant women) or using damp loo paper. Try a witch hazel compress, as above. If you keep bleeding, or if the pain is not relieved easily, don't be embarrassed to seek help. This is a very common problem indeed.

Constipation

Unfortunately, because the bowel absorbs more water in pregnancy, and because the movements of the gut are reduced, constipation is a problem experienced by most pregnant women. It is important to overcome it if you can, as straining exacerbates problems with piles if you have them. Try to take more fluids, particularly water and fruit juices (avoiding tea, which tends to constipate), and increase your intake of fruit, vegetables and fibre-rich foods. Although you may think that munching bran, or indeed putting bran on your cereal may help, suddenly adding lots of bran to your diet can make things worse, giving you a bloated stomach. Snacking on dried fruits, e.g. prunes and apricots, is usually helpful. Iron tablets tend to cause constipation, so if you are taking them ask your GP whether they are strictly necessary. A brisk walk or other exercise every day will also help. Whilst there are some very mild laxatives that can be taken safely in pregnancy, in general you should avoid them as they can start off contractions.

Morning Sickness

As many pregnant women discover to their cost, pregnancy sickness seldom occurs only in the morning. There are all sorts of theories about its cause but, surprisingly perhaps for such a common problem, none has yet been proven. It is known that stress and lifestyle play some part – it is least prevalent amongst Eskimos, for instance.

Let's deal with the old wives' tales first. You will often be told that pregnancy sickness is 'good', sometimes by well-meaning GPs, and that it means that pregnancy is well established. Whilst it is true that those who report vomiting to their GP are less likely to miscarry, or have a premature or stillborn child, the converse (that no morning sickness is a bad sign) is false. You may also be told, in complete contradiction, that excessive morning sickness (hyperemesis gravidarum) is linked with unhealthy pregnancy. Whilst it is the case that one or two conditions are linked to hyperemesis (such as hydatidiform mole (see Chapter 10), these are rare (molar pregnancy occurs in 1 in 2000 pregnancies and excessive sickness isn't always a symptom by any means; by contrast hyperemesis occurs in 1 in 100 pregnancies). Because it is said (incorrectly) that high levels of female hormones are responsible for morning sickness, it is said (incorrectly) that you are more likely to have bad morning sickness if you are carrying a girl. I wouldn't order the pink curtains on the strength of this one.

The thing that will probably worry you most, especially if you are losing weight and existing on nothing much more than a couple of dry biscuits a day, is how the baby is faring. You may feel, particularly if your pregnancy was unplanned and you didn't have the opportunity of a period of sustained and deliberate 'good things' eating before conception, that your baby is impossibly disadvantaged by your condition. All the available evidence is heartwarming. Even in those women who have the severest hyperemesis, pregnancy outcome is usually good with no added risk to mother, unborn baby or newly delivered baby.

For most women, morning sickness will disappear by about 16 weeks. For an unfortunate few, vomiting will continue throughout pregnancy. There was a very effective drug, Debendox; however, this has now been removed from the market because of concerns about possible malformation in babies despite very strong evidence to the contrary. The drug was prescribed to about a third of pregnancies, and if it really was responsible for malformations, one would have expected a reduction when it was withdrawn in June 1983. This has not been the case. In fact, as Iain Chalmers and others point out in *Effective Care in Pregnancy and Childbirth* (Oxford University Press, 1990), 'if an overall congenital malformation incidence of 3.5 per cent at delivery is assumed, then exposure to Debendox will have occurred in over one million babies born with congenital malformation by chance alone. In the inevitable search for what may have produced her child's malformations, it is not surprising that many mothers implicated Debendox, and perhaps prompted by over eager lawyers, some chose to sue.'

Antihistamines, which seem to be effective, but whose safety has not been as extensively studied as that of Debendox, are now being prescribed. They have side effects such as drowsiness and blurred vision and although they are generally considered safe there has been no major epidemiological study to look for teratogenic effects.

Which leave you with what? Management is the first option. There are probably some things which make you feel acutely nauseous – the smell of coffee (something I loved prior to and after pregnancy) was what did it to me – so enlist your partner's help to try and avoid contact with the things that you know set it off. Fried food and roast dinners are two other particular culprits, so perhaps this is the time to go for salads and casseroles. You may also become acutely sensitive to some smells. I've heard some very curious examples in my time of this – one lady said that the smell of a particular brand of soap made her heave when pregnant. Her husband inadvertently bought some and she could tell, when he walked through the front door, that he had a bar of 'that stuff' in a carrier bag, although it was wrapped and she could not see it. One of the most difficult problems is when you work closely with someone whose heavy perfume suddenly makes you very nauseous. Getting out for a brisk walk in the fresh air can make you feel better, but you do have to be quite bold to tell someone that their perfume makes you feel sick. Such smells are frequently encountered in squashed masses of people, as found on tubes, buses and trains, where that and the effect of the motion may be overwhelming. Again, management is the key. If you can possibly start later so that you travel outside the rush-hour peak, do so.

The other trick is to start the day slowly. Get your partner to bring you tea in bed first thing. Chew a plain biscuit (like a Rich Tea) and get up by degrees. Don't let yourself become hungry (when blood sugar levels drop between meals, the feelings of nausea seem to be at their worst). Frequent snacks seem to help. Bland food is often recommended, but sometimes strong tastes and flavours make women feel better – it is a condition where only trial and error can identify what is best avoided in your case. If you possibly can, get someone else to prepare food for you and avoid lots of cooking. If you already have children, this may not be wildly practical, but you are hereby given permission to chuck the superwoman apron away and give them ready prepared meals for a while. You may feel that you are copping out by doing this, but who cares – having frozen lasagne instead of homemade for a couple of months isn't going to kill anyone. And if you feel less sick, it's worth doing.

A lot of women find that sipping fizzy drinks is helpful. Try to avoid the sugary ones and go for the diet versions, or for fruit juice diluted with sparkling water. Another remedy is ginger, which is famous for its anti-emetic properties. You can take it as tablets, as an infusion made from fresh shredded root, as crystallised ginger or even as ginger beer.

7

Medical Complications in Pregnancy

'When they said that a smear test was routine, it never crossed my mind that I might have a positive result. When it did come back positive, I went hot and cold and spent the next three days crying my eyes out. There was nothing anywhere about abnormal smears in pregnancy. When they said that they wouldn't treat it in pregnancy, I had these dreadful visions of my husband, pushing a pram at my funeral. I had colposcopy when I was about six months pregnant and although they reassured me, I didn't stop worrying until I'd had Kylie and had had laser treatment. It wrecked my pregnancy and I'd advise anyone planning pregnancy to make sure that they've had a smear recently because then it won't mean going through what I went through.'

'No one ever told me that it was possible to bleed all through pregnancy.'

'I had a haemorrhage when I was 29 weeks. It was the most frightening thing that's ever happened to me.'

'I spotted all the time and then discovered I had a low-lying placenta. I spent several weeks in hospital, but I felt like a complete fraud because I was so healthy. I moaned all the time about being in there until I started to haemorrhage and then I just thanked my lucky stars that

*I was in hospital, and not at home, 35 miles away, with
just a toddler and a nutty collie on hand to help.'*

*'It's no good people telling you that bleeding doesn't
harm the baby. You still worry about it. After all the
bleeding I'd had I'd convinced myself I'd have this pale
thin baby but I had a 9 lbs 3 oz hulk instead.'*

Abnormal Smear in Pregnancy

Almost all pregnant women will have a cervical smear taken
during pregnancy unless you've been having regular smears
anyhow – usually at the booking visit. This is not because
pregnant women are at greater risk of cervical cancer. It is
simply that pregnancy is an unrivalled opportunity to take
smears from all women, rather than just those who turn up for
smear testing.

The important point to make from the outset is that
cervical cancer is a totally preventable cancer. Rather in the
way that cinemas used to run trailers for 'the big film', so your
cervix obligingly runs up warning flags before the 'big feature'
makes an appearance. The presence of such flags does not
mean you have cancer – it just means that you need to watch,
wait and sometimes take action to prevent cervical cancer
occurring. Most of this 'action' can safely be deferred until
after the birth.

There is no evidence whatsoever that conversion from
warning flags to actual cancer occurs because of pregnancy.

Briefly, your vagina is lined with tough, flat cells. Your
womb is lined with tall, delicate cells. These two types of cell
meet on your cervix, the gristly plug at the bottom of your
womb. If warning flags are flying, they will fly first in the no-

man's-land (the so-called transformation zone) between these two types of cell. When a smear is taken, cells are deliberately taken from this no-man's-land. The first 'grade' of warning flag is called CIN I (CIN stands for cervical intraepithelial neoplasia). Think of it rather like a flag warning of an uneven pavement ahead. Many (about 60 per cent of CIN I abnormalities resolve spontaneously (as if someone had gone round in the night and relaid that pavement properly). In CIN II, there are more flags flying, for the pavement ahead has quite a few cracked paving stones, and some of them are laid a bit higgledy-piggledy. It might resolve itself but this would be unusual. In CIN III, even more flags fly, for there is almost no order to the pavement ahead – in fact it looks more like crazy paving. CIN III will definitely progress to cancer unless treated. One word of warning; sometimes CIN III is written in notes as 'carcinoma in situ'. Be reassured; you still haven't got cancer, for CIN I, II and III are all pre-cancerous changes, not cancer itself.

Such cell changes are not, in general, speedy. In fact they may take up to twenty years. However, for a minority of women there does seem to be a type of fast-track cell change. Doctors are still searching for information which will tell them which abnormal smears are likely to 'fast track' and which are not. Until such information is available, they must treat every abnormal smear as a potential fast tracker. Thus, if you have a mildly abnormal smear in pregnancy you may have a repeat smear every month to check that the situation isn't getting worse, but many hospitals would want you to have your cervix examined with a colposcope.

A colposcope is a device which both illuminates and magnifies the cervix. It is not uncomfortable to have colposcopy, although it is a mite undignified (you lie rather like a stranded beetle with your legs in stirrups) but frankly, compared to giving birth, it's a cinch. Diagnosis with colposcopy is particularly accurate in pregnancy because the cervix changes colour, becoming darker, which serves to accentuate the differences between normal and abnormal cells. Most gynaecologists would want to take a biopsy – a small sample of tissue – from your cervix just to double-check that they were not missing an early case of cancer. All this sounds horribly alarming. You might imagine for a start that it would cause a miscarriage; in fact this is very unlikely. Bleeding is a theoretical concern, but again the risks are very low. If CIN is found, the usual procedure is to repeat the colposcopy between 24 and 34 weeks of pregnancy, and then again at 8 weeks post-partum, and to then arrange for treatment in the normal way (i.e. with a laser, cryosurgery, etc.) about three or four months after the birth.

If early signs of an invading cancer were found, a cone biopsy – in which a cone of tissue, including the abnormal bit, is removed from the cervix – might be indicated. This isn't the easiest of procedures for the gynaecologist, but the good news is that 9 out of 10 women will still have the healthy baby they want, even if the cone biopsy is undertaken relatively early in pregnancy. Eight out of 10 women will go to term, despite having had a cone biopsy.

There are conflicting emotions about abnormal smears and their treatment in pregnancy. On one hand, you are acutely aware of your baby and don't want to do anything which might be endangering. I hope that I've shown you that even if it got to cone biopsy – which is an extreme – your baby still has all the odds stacked in his or her favour. On the other hand, you will be pressured by your gynaecologist, your family and above all your partner to take action with regard to yourself. Having a biopsy seems to be a balance of risks – you are reassuring yourself and those who love you, but leaving any action until after the baby is born when you absolutely must have further investigation and treatment if necessary.

Finally, and I say it simply because this came up in the survey – from a woman who had an abnormal smear and thought she was going to die as a result – 85 per cent of women who die of cervical cancer have never had a smear. Only 1 in 5,000 women has an invasive cancer of the cervix (true cervical cancer) diagnosed in pregnancy. The fact that your condition has been picked up, rather than left to become more advanced, automatically gives you a more than very good chance of total recovery. By all means write a will now that you are thinking in terms of a family, but don't do it on account of cervical cancer.

Bleeding in Later Pregnancy

PLACENTA PRAEVIA

Women having ultrasound scans are very often told that they have a low-lying placenta. And in the next breath, the doctor or ultrasonographer says that it may be nothing to worry about because the placenta is likely to move. This causes a great deal of confusion because, quite rightly, women's impression of the placenta is that it is firmly anchored in one place. The thought of a peripatetic placenta is a bit spooky. Let me explain.

Potentially, the entire lining of the womb is receptive to the fertilised egg. However, the upper portion of the womb has a rich blood supply and the embryo normally implants here. But a good many embryos (probably about 30 per cent) implant in the lower segment, near the canal that leads through the cervix to the vagina, the cervical os (pronounced 'oss'). All but 3 per cent of these will 'migrate'. They don't actually move, of course, but as the womb grows, the placenta is pulled upwards. In addition, the chorionic villi, with little fingers of placental tissue that anchor the placenta to the womb lining, have the ability, some people believe, to grow in one area and remain dormant in another, thus encouraging growth of the placenta higher up the womb than lower. If you are told you have a low-lying placenta, the odds are overwhelmingly in favour of it 'moving', thus causing you no further worries. 'Low-lying placenta' is a very over-diagnosed condition and if you are told this in early pregnancy, you should firmly ignore it, secure in the knowledge that only 3 per cent of women with this diagnosis will actually have a placenta which is so abnormally placed that it will require caesarean section to deliver the baby. A second scan is normally required to tell doctors what they knew anyway – i.e. that the placenta has indeed 'moved'. In the meantime, had you not read this, you would have been caused a great deal of unnecessary anxiety.

If the placenta continues to lie very close to, or even over the cervical os, it is called placenta praevia. The main concern is haemorrhage. The main symptom of placenta praevia is painless spotting of bright red blood in an otherwise normal pregnancy, which usually occurs in the third trimester. If there are no such symptoms, there is a 90 per cent chance of it changing to a normal placenta before delivery, but frequent observations with scan will be required to check this.

There are different 'grades' of placenta praevia, depending on how much of the cervical os is covered.

As pregnancy advances, the Braxton Hicks contractions (the pretend contractions that your womb practises during pregnancy) cause the lower part of the womb to thin, in preparation for labour. This means that some portions of the abnormally positioned placenta separate from the womb wall. Because the blood is not trapped behind the placenta, it is fresh and bright. The first episode of bleeding is usually minor, is accompanied by no pain and is relatively late in pregnancy (after 20 weeks). Because the bottom half of the womb isn't able to contract as efficiently as the top half, any bleeding involving the lower section tends to be dramatic. Second bleeds are not usually as minor, and the condition is treacherous in that bleeding is very unpredictable indeed. Very often the bleeding is unprovoked, but sometimes it follows lovemaking. You should expect to be admitted to hospital even though your due date may be some time off and, because of the unpredictable nature of this condition, to have to stay there.

When you get to hospital, the priority will be to cross match your blood and to arrange for sufficient blood to be available just in case you do haemorrhage. Unless your blood loss has been severe, most hospitals adopt a 'watch and wait' approach, in the hope that they can get you to 36 or 37 weeks before delivering the baby by an elective caesarean. A caesarean is usually necessary. This is not only because the baby's exit from the womb is effectively blocked, but also because as the cervix dilates more and more of the placenta will come away from the womb, causing very severe haemorrhage from the arteries which have been exposed and also, of course, cutting off the blood supply, and hence the oxygen supply, to the baby. However, vaginal delivery may still be possible with a grade 1 placenta praevia. The one thing that will not be undertaken, unless you are in an operating theatre with full transfusion facilities immediately at hand, is a vaginal examination, since it can provoke serious bleeding. Vaginal ultrasound, although it is 100 per cent accurate in diagnosing placenta praevia, is unlikely to be used for the same reason.

Normally, the senior consultant would supervise a caesarean section for placenta praevia. If you think about it, the placenta, especially if it is stuck on the front of the lower womb, is just where the section incision would ordinarily be made. In addition women who have had a previous caesarean, for another indication altogether, are more at risk of the placenta sticking fast to the womb wall (placenta acreta), which is another reason for the section being supervised by the consultant. There is still a substantial risk of haemorrhage. Although it may all sound a bit alarming, this is in fact a good news story. If the pregnancy goes to 36 or 37 weeks, the outcome for the baby is very good indeed. For the mother there is drama, and quite a lot of blood may be lost at delivery, but the outcome is also very good, in contrast to the situation at the turn of the century, when placenta praevia was regularly the cause of death of both mother and baby. The main concerns for the baby are those that surround all babies that are born too soon (see the chapter on prematurity), which is why the watch and wait approach is so important.

CAUSES

The causes of placenta praevia are obscure. There are a number of things which predispose to placenta praevia, which is not the same thing at all as saying that they are the cause. They include having had many children previously, increasing age, multiple pregnancy and previous caesarean section.

COPING

It is very difficult to cope with a crisis pregnancy like this, partly because you feel so out of control and partly because when medical emergency threatens, your feelings are the last things that anyone thinks about. Of course you wouldn't want it any other way, but it may make you feel that you are an uninvolved onlooker. Extended bed rest in hospital and the resultant separation from family and your partner can take its toll on even the most loving of relationships. And just because you have a placenta praevia, doesn't mean that you will feel unwell. In fact, you may feel blooming and this makes extended bed rest very hard to bear, with you feeling a complete fraud.

Trying Again

Placenta praevia has a small recurrence rate – about 5 per cent – but you may nevertheless feel very anxious about another pregnancy. A prolonged spell in hospital is bad enough when it's just you and your partner, but trying to cope when you also have a toddler to care for is very difficult. Nevertheless the odds are stacked in your favour.

PLACENTAL ABRUPTION

In about 1 to 1.5 per cent of pregnancies, the placenta becomes partially or totally separated (abrupted) from the wall of the womb. This can happen at any stage of pregnancy but is more common towards the end. Unlike placenta praevia, the placenta is normally sited but becomes separated because of bleeding between it and the womb lining. The effect of this separation is to reduce, or even cut off the oxygen supply to the baby, although abruption severe enough to cause the baby's death immediately is a rare event (1 in 500).

Sometimes the pool of blood behind the placenta tracks upwards, towards the top of the womb. This means that the blood doesn't escape via the vagina, but continues to pool. This is called a concealed abruption. Concealed bleeding is more hazardous, simply because diagnosis may be delayed.

Haemoglobin, the blood pigment, may seep into the muscle of the womb, turning it a bluish colour and making it look very bruised. There may be intense abdominal pain, but if the placenta is stuck to the back wall of the womb, there could be lower back pain. If there has only been a small bleed, there may be pain over the site of the bleed. If the pool of blood extends downwards, bleeding will be evident via the vagina, with the blood being a very dark colour.

Ultrasound scanning cannot help, detecting only 2 per cent of abruptions, which means that placental abruption has to be diagnosed principally from clinical signs which, from the above, you will appreciate are diverse and confusing. If the abruption is small, rest and luck may ensure that the pregnancy continues. However, even a small abruption can cause premature labour and the baby may be born too early to survive. With a severe abruption, an immediate caesarean section is undertaken to try and save both mother and baby. Another problem of a severe abruption is that the pool of blood behind the placenta begins to clot. Because there is such a large volume of blood, this has the potential to use up all the blood's clotting factors. This means that when the baby is delivered, bleeding from the placental site doesn't stop because there are no clotting agents left. This frightening and desperate emergency is called disseminated intravascular coagulopathy (DIC), and requires extensive specialist transfusion services. Thankfully, it happens very rarely because doctors are aware of the dangers. It does mean that you will get completely taken over by high tech medicine. Accept it.

Coping

There is no disguising the fact that placental abruption is a grave emergency. About a third of the babies involved in placental abruption cases will die. Without specialist care, the mother would die as well, particularly where there is a coagulation problem. Maternal mortality is now very rare indeed. Physical recovery may take some time, but emotional recovery may take a great deal longer, especially, of course, if your baby died. About 15 per cent of stillbirths are caused by placental abruption. There is acute sadness and loss, which is compounded by feeling very weak. For your partner, who may have been far more aware than you of the life-threatening crisis you faced, there may be overwhelming and conflicting emotions. Guilt perhaps that you were his prime concern and not the baby; relief that you've come through it; delayed shock and again, great sadness and grief. Your baby may have come through this ordeal but be in special care, especially if the delivery was premature. As with all acute medical emergencies, the full impact of what you have both faced may not hit you for some time.

Causes

Little is known about the causes of placental abruption. Once again there are a series of predisposing factors, such as smoking, low social class and maternal age. Abruption is a common cause of fetal loss in the Third World, leading to suggestions that poverty and malnutrition play an important role. However, a suggestion that it is due to folate or other vitamin deficiency has fallen out of favour since giving supplements to women with a previous abruption did not reduce the incidence thereafter. Abruption has been persistently linked with high blood pressure and this would certainly seem a logical association. There is some dispute about whether high blood pressure follows the abruption or causes it, but it seems that there is an increased risk for those women with pre-eclampsia.

As you might expect, placental abruption can follow a direct blow to the abdomen, either from assault or more commonly following injury in a car collision. Findings from California implicated seatbelts as a cause of abruption in those women who survived a car crash whilst wearing a seatbelt. On the other hand, pregnant women who don't wear seatbelts get thrown through the windscreen and are even more likely to suffer abruption as a result of impact with the road. Finally, abruption has followed snake bite (just in case you should come across a snake whilst shopping in Mothercare).

Trying Again

The risk of abruption in a subsequent pregnancy is about the same as that for placenta praevia – 6 per cent. If you have a second abruption, the recurrence rate rises to 25 per cent. This suggests that there might be an underlying abnormality in the womb or in its blood supply, although no one has ever documented what this might be – and in any case you can't alter your physiology. The principle preventive measure is to stop smoking (a reduction of risk of 23 per cent). If high blood pressure has been associated with the abruption, then anti-hypertensive drugs may be suggested. Despite there being no strong evidence about its efficacy, some doctors will give folates in a subsequent pregnancy. If the abruption occurred late in pregnancy, a decision may be taken to induce the baby two weeks or so beforehand in another pregnancy.

8

Miscarriage

'I wish I'd known how common miscarriage was.'

'The GP told me that I was being overcautious – after three miscarriages.'

'I wish I'd known I'd get to the end, then I wouldn't have worried quite so much.'

'If only I'd known that 1 in 6 pregnancies miscarry, I don't think I would have felt so miserable and alone.'

Most people would be surprised to know that of every 100 pregnancies, between 10 and 20 will end in miscarriage. Miscarriage is a very common event indeed. In fact, it may be even more common than we imagine. Using very sensitive pregnancy tests, it can be shown that up to 75 per cent of all conceptions will fail, most before we are even aware that we are pregnant, with the remainder occurring mostly in the early months of pregnancy.

These days, very few women consciously set out to have a big family. In consequence each of our pregnancies carries a heavy investment, in terms of our hopes, our emotions and our aspirations about how we see ourselves and our families in the future. Despite the fact that there can be few of us who do not know someone who has had a miscarriage, we expect our pregnancies to go to term, and what is more, to have healthy babies. Having a miscarriage challenges all our expectations. Guilt, a sense of failure, confusion, disappointment and grief are just some of the emotions faced not only by women experiencing miscarriage, but by their partners too.

Before explaining some of the causes of miscarriage, it is worth clearing up some of the misunderstanding, and indeed hurt, caused by the medical terminology used in connection with miscarriage. Firstly, the legal definition of miscarriage has recently been changed and is now used to describe any event which expels the baby from the womb before 24 weeks of pregnancy (and not 28 weeks of pregnancy as it used to be).

There are a whole series of medical phrases, which describe the way in which a miscarriage occurs rather than the cause. You may hear spontaneous abortion, threatened abortion, incomplete abortion, missed abortion, inevitable abortion and also recurrent abortion. Women find doctors' use of the word abortion distressing. For them, abortion means unwanted babies and the deliberate ending of a pregnancy, not the miserable end to a much wanted pregnancy. You may feel concerned about the use of the phrase abortion in your notes, fearing perhaps that it may be misunderstood. It won't be. What we would call an abortion is written medically either as 'induced abortion' or alternatively 'termination of pregnancy (TOP)'.

For spontaneous abortion just read miscarriage. A 'threatened miscarriage' is used to describe a situation where there is bleeding and perhaps some pain. Although 'threatened' sounds as if the baby is in danger, in reality the bleeding often settles down and many women will then go on to have healthy babies, despite this fright. When bleeding is heavy to severe (similar to a normal period), the cervix is dilating and there are cramp-like pains, a miscarriage is termed 'inevitable'. A complete abortion simply describes a situation in which all three elements of pregnancy – sac, placenta and baby, the so-called 'products of conception' – have come away. Incomplete abortion means that, despite the miscarriage, some material still remains in the womb. A dilatation and curettage operation (D&C) may be necessary to remove it, as otherwise bleeding may continue.

Missed abortion describes the type of miscarriage where the baby has failed to develop properly and has then died, but is not lost immediately. There may be some spotting of blood, and the woman usually starts to feel less and less pregnant, losing such signs of pregnancy as breast tenderness and nausea. Normally the combination of these symptoms would suggest the need for a scan, which will quickly reveal that the baby is dead. Sometimes, at earlier stages of pregnancy, the baby may be completely resorbed by the mother's body, leaving an empty sac. If you have seen the baby on an earlier scan, seeing an empty sac on scan can be quite a shock.

It is not known why fetal death in some instances is quickly followed by miscarriage, but in others miscarriage is delayed. Eventually, in these situations, a miscarriage may occur. However, most women would prefer not to wait for this to happen, but would rather have a D&C immediately. In fact, a D&C is essential sooner rather than later. This is because after a certain length of time (about a month) the dead material inside the womb could provoke a coagulation defect (where inappropriate clotting in minor vessels occurs, which uses up all the blood clotting factors). If this were to happen, catastrophic haemorrhage would occur when the womb was emptied.

Recurrent abortion is a history of three or more consecutive miscarriages. Sometimes this is also called habitual abortion. Finally, you may also hear the phrase 'blighted ovum' or 'anembryonic pregnancy'. These two phrases mean the same thing and describe a pregnancy in which a placenta and sac has formed but no baby. All you will see on scan is an empty sac. Because pregnancy hormones are produced by the placenta, you will feel pregnant, even though there has never been a baby. This type of pregnancy can end in any of the ways described above.

An 'early' miscarriage is one which occurs before 16 weeks. A late miscarriage can occur up to 24 weeks. Some people argue that pregnancy loss is the same whether the baby is at 8 weeks gestation, 18 weeks, or 38 weeks. Whilst I go some way down this particular road, there is a difference, I think, both in the physical and emotional experience, between a miscarriage at 8 weeks and a stillbirth at 38 weeks. But as ever, there are no absolutes.

One word of caution; as I have indicated, the majority of conceptions will fail, mostly before women are even aware that they are pregnant. Until recently, the fact that women had been pregnant in this way – a so-called biochemical pregnancy – was only demonstrable in hospital laboratories. Now the same technology is available over the counter in any chemist. Pregnancy testing kits can be used on the first day of a missed period. You may well get a positive result, and then have a period a couple of days later. Is this a miscarriage? I think the answer to this is a firm no.

Another confusion created by pregnancy testing was brought home to me recently by a lady who telephoned me in some distress. She had had a positive pregnancy test and then, after experiencing bleeding a couple of days later, had a scan, only to be told that the baby had been dead for a week or more. How, she wondered, could the test have been positive when the baby was dead? The basis of testing is beta hCG, a hormone which is produced by the placenta, not the baby. Thus testing is based on the likely presence of a placenta, not a baby.

Symptoms

If you talk to women about their experience of miscarriage, one thing is immediately clear. There is no one pattern of miscarriage; even bleeding isn't a universal experience, and a miscarriage can occur quite dramatically with no prior symptoms whatsoever. Even in those who have had the misfortune to have several miscarriages, each one may occur in a different way.

BLEEDING

Bleeding is usually the first symptom. A general rule of thumb is that if the bleeding is equivalent to a normal period loss, the pregnancy is unlikely to be successful – but even so, there are some pregnancies which come through such dramas with flying colours. Bleeding in pregnancy is more common than you might think, and miscarriage is certainly not inevitable. In fact about half of all those women who experience bleeding in pregnancy will go on to have a healthy baby. It is of course possible that the bleeding is nothing to do with pregnancy at all; small lesions of the vagina and cervix and cervical polyps can all be the source of bleeding.

Because our experience with blood is that it comes from an injury of some sort, we assume, if we see blood during pregnancy, that it must have come from the baby, or be hurting the baby in some way. However, it is quite possible for bleeding to occur in early pregnancy which does not compromise the baby at all. For instance, when the fertilised egg burrows into the side of the womb, a small amount of womb lining comes to lie over the top of it. This bit of lining dies off and is then shed, usually between 12 and 25 days after fertilisation. Another source of bleeding is that part of the womb lining which is not yet obscured by the developing sac. The only way I can think of describing what I mean by this is for you to think of one blown-up balloon (the womb), with another, deflated one (the sac containing the baby) inside it. If you inflated the inside balloon, there would be a point where it was touching some of the outer balloon, but not all of it. A similar situation exists in the womb in early pregnancy, and for some women it is possible, if their hormonal environment is appropriate, for there to be some bleeding from this bit of lining. Coincidence sometimes dictates that this occurs at times when they would have had a period, i.e. at 4, 8 and 12 weeks. Probably arising from this, there is a myth that miscarriage is most likely to occur at the time that you would have had a period and I often hear it said that women should be particularly careful at this time. This has no foundation in science at all.

Another source of bleeding which, although it has greater significance than the above, can also be of little consequence, is minor bleeding behind the placenta. The placenta is pretty well anchored into the womb lining, but there may be small sections along its edge which work loose exposing blood vessels. Bleeding will then occur in the gap between the placenta and the wall of the womb. If the bleeding isn't too great, it will form clots and then seal itself off – which is why you sometimes see fresh red blood which then becomes brownish and finally stops.

If you have had a threatened miscarriage, and if, after a little while, during which time you have had some bed rest, it has settled down, there is usually someone in your life who will say something particularly helpful on the lines of 'miscarriages were meant to be, you're cheating nature'. The inference is that miscarriage happens because babies are abnormal and that because you 'stopped' your miscarriage, your baby is likely to be abnormal in some way. I hope from what I've said about the different sources of bleeding that I have convinced you that this is untrue. In addition, you should note that even amongst women who have pain accompanied by quite heavy bleeding, one in three will overcome this initial problem and have a normal pregnancy thereafter. The crucial question is, are their babies normal? The answer is reassuring. A recent large survey revealed that women who had experienced bleeding in early pregnancy were no more likely to have an abnormal baby than women who had no such problems – so stop worrying about this one.

In contrast to the above, where miscarriage simply threatens, in cases where a threatened miscarriage proceeds to an inevitable miscarriage, bleeding has usually started only after the baby has died.

Having a Miscarriage

You should tell someone if you think you are having or have had a miscarriage, even if it is a very early one. This is particularly important if you know you have rhesus negative blood, as you will need to have a shot of Anti D within seventy-two hours of the miscarriage to prevent the possible build-up of antibodies, which potentially might be harmful to a subsequent pregnancy. Since many women do not know their blood group when they first become pregnant, telling your GP should either precipitate some burrowing in your notes (it might be recorded somewhere) or a blood test to quickly establish your blood group. If you, like 90 per cent of the population, have rhesus positive blood, you need have no further worries. Neither should you worry if you have rhesus negative blood, because once you have had anti-D, your next pregnancy is unlikely to be affected by rhesus problems.

Most women, faced with cramping pain and bleeding in early pregnancy, will telephone their GPs. If bleeding is heavy, or if bleeding is heavy with pain, expect to be referred to hospital. There are several reasons for this; an ultrasound scan will indicate immediately whether the baby is alive or dead. If the baby is dead, there is no point in prolonging the agony of waiting for the inevitable to happen. Most women would prefer to get it over, and have a D & C or, as it so often seems to be called today, an ERPOC – which stands for Evacuation of the Retained Products of Conception (a truly horrible phrase in my view) – which is normally undertaken under general anaesthetic. Another reason for wanting to be in hospital is simply fear of the unknown and wondering how you are going to cope at home. However, whilst hospital admission is essential for later loss, women in early pregnancy may prefer to stay at home, feeling that going to hospital will change something that is personal and private into a public, medical event.

Some doctors feel that all women who have had a miscarriage should be admitted to hospital for a D & C on the grounds that all tissue might not have come away, therefore predisposing to infection. However, in the vast majority of cases, the womb empties itself very efficiently and many GPs, and quite a few hospital consultants as well, would argue that a D & C is quite unnecessary for most women. The situations where a D & C may be required are in incomplete miscarriages and particularly for missed miscarriage cases, for the reasons I explained earlier. However, if this is your situation and you feel that you would rather let nature take its own course, you can probably leave it for a week or ten days in the hope that the miscarriage will occur naturally. But after this time you will need to consider a D & C.

As I have indicated, a GP's course of action when there is pain and heavy bleeding is fairly clearcut, but for spotting or scant bleeding without pain a wide range of reactions is possible. Some GPs will advise bed rest, some will advise to continue as normal, although avoiding heavy tasks such as shopping and lifting, some will be positively unhelpful and uninterested and say things like 'What do you expect me to do about it?' Whilst this sort of view is distressing, it articulates the impotence the medical profession feels in this situation. There are no medical miracle wands that they can wave. Miscarriage, however, is unpleasant and upsetting and GPs and other health professionals can do much to make women feel that they are supported and cared for, even though there may be little they can do medically.

Miscarriages are not, in general, clearcut events. There is often a period of time when you think it might happen, but don't know for sure. You worry and wait, sometimes only for your worst fears to be realised. Whilst many GPs advocate a 'wait and see' strategy with bleeding in early pregnancy, this creates dreadful uncertainty and it is intolerable, I think, for this uncertainty to be allowed to continue for any length of time when a scan can, in most cases, quickly resolve whether the pregnancy is viable or not. Probably the most helpful thing your GP can do is refer you promptly for a scan. I have said that about 50 per cent of pregnancies complicated by threatened miscarriage have a successful outcome. If a fetal heartbeat can be identified on scan, outcome is successful in 90 per cent of cases.

Bed rest is very frequent advice. In fact, it may be your first reaction too. It has the great advantage of not being harmful, being cheap and easy to dispense, and it also makes you feel you are doing something positive to help. Unfortunately the results of the only study on this gave no support to the view that bed rest reduces the risk of miscarriage after bleeding occurs in early pregnancy. Some women who experienced bleeding in early pregnancy swear it was bed rest that got them through their pregnancies, but logic would say that bed rest will do nothing to prevent the inevitable and that in a substantial proportion of pregnancies complicated by early bleeding the baby is already dead. Prolonged bed rest can be very disruptive to home and family life, too. The best advice is probably to do what you feel is appropriate for you. If you decide to carry on as normal, then it makes sense to lessen your load if you can, not because there is any evidence to show that hard work or worry or stress will finally tip the balance and precipitate a miscarriage, but because if you have taken things a bit easy, at least if you do have a miscarriage you will not have a stick with which to beat yourself emotionally.

Having a miscarriage at home can be alarming. You may pass quite large clots of blood, particularly when on the loo. There may be a recognisable baby, depending on the stage of pregnancy, but there may not, usually because it has already died and begun to decompose. Women usually need and want to know what they have lost. If they do not see it, they may become anxious and upset, imagining something far worse than reality. What you do with this material depends very much on how you feel about it. If there is no recognisable baby, some people would just flush the loo and have done with it; some people would prefer to bury such material as there is in the garden, perhaps beneath a tree; some would prefer to ring the hospital and ask if they could dispose of it. Some hospitals are sensitive about this, and some not.

Sometimes it is difficult for them to be practical (like suggesting the material be brought in a plastic box or bag) without the advice sounding incongruous and heartless. Most hospitals have strict guidelines on the sensitive disposal of miscarriage material. Actually, I'm having a hard time just writing the word 'disposal' but, try as I might, I cannot think of a more sympathetic word. Forgive me.

TREATMENT

As I have indicated, once miscarriage threatens, there is no specific treatment. However, that hasn't stopped a great many doctors over a great many years offering injections of various hormones as an antidote to threatened miscarriage. Progestogen or hCG injections have not been shown to reduce the risk of miscarriage. In fact, tender loving care (extra care in pregnancy, frequency scans, access to a twenty-four-hour helpline) seems to be the most effective treatment yet devised; but no amount of TLC will restore a pregnancy that has already ended. Having a doctor who is on your side, however, and who treats you sympathetically and with respect, helps immeasurably. You will find advice about treatment designed to prevent miscarriages caused by specific problems later in this chapter.

For early miscarriages, hospital admission followed by ERPOC may be appropriate. Following an incomplete miscarriage, you may again have to be admitted to hospital for ERPOC, but this can often be undertaken as a day case. For later miscarriages hospital admission is essential. For some women, the investigations prompted by an episode of bleeding may reveal that the baby has died. Whilst an ERPOC is appropriate for early pregnancy loss, after about 16 weeks this is no longer possible (because of the possibility of damaging your cervix with adverse consequences for future pregnancies) and labour will need to be induced. This can be a distressing experience, but hopefully the hospital staff will handle it with care and sensitivity.

If this is the case, you should ask all the questions you want, including those you may fear asking such as 'What will the baby look like?' It is not always the case that the baby will have decomposed. You don't have to see the baby when it is born, but you may find that it helps you to come to terms with your loss if you can say goodbye in your own way.

Just because this is not full term labour does not mean that pain relief is not appropriate – it is, if you feel that you want it. Some women prefer to be very much aware of this experience; others feel that pain relief helps them feel more in control of what is happening. Also this is a rare instance of being able to put your needs ahead of those of the baby, so the normal considerations of effect of analgesia on the baby do not apply.

After a Miscarriage

Expect to bleed for about two weeks following a miscarriage. You should use sanitary towels rather than tampons because of the risk of infection and you should avoid lovemaking until the bleeding has ceased, for the same reason. If your bleeding seems to be increasing rather than decreasing, or if it starts to smell offensive, seek help from your GP immediately.

COPING

Before going on to the all important 'why', it is important to talk about how to cope with a miscarriage, because it is so often a miserable experience which may leave you feeling inadequate and unhappy. Doctors can be horribly insensitive. On the one hand it is important that they reassure you that miscarriages are the most common sorts of pregnancy loss, but on the other hand they ought to understand that grief and loss are common reactions too. Miscarriage in the first three months is very much a silent loss, not only because you and your partner may be the only ones to know about it, but also because you often have no concrete memories about the pregnancy. If you have a miscarriage, an early scan picture can suddenly become immensely precious. Few people offer as much sympathy as is really needed, simply because they do not understand its impact; nor can they understand how you can have become so attached to a baby you never saw, and sometimes didn't even feel moving. People may say things which you find very hurtful, although they mean to be kind: 'You can always have another one' (yes, probably, but it was that baby you wanted); or 'It was probably for the best' (it might have been, but it's no consolation).

You will probably experience a bewildering range of emotions. There may initially be a sense of relief, particularly if you went through a period of uncertainty about the pregnancy. You may feel shocked and unable to believe what has happened. You may feel completely helpless because you were powerless to prevent it happening. You may feel angry that this has happened to you and take out that anger on the doctor, or your partner. You may feel guilty, thinking that you were responsible for your miscarriage – if only you hadn't gone late-night shopping, if only you hadn't lifted that box. A common feeling is failure – after all, here is life's most basic function and yet you couldn't do it – you and about 500,000 other women in Britain each year, that is.

You will suddenly find that the world is full of pregnant women, that the papers are full of smiling people with babies, and as if this weren't enough, your best friend will ring to say that she is pregnant. It all seems very unfair and you may just want to hibernate and avoid everybody. I know that I felt that I could cope; provided, that is, people didn't start being very sympathetic — that finished me off completely. All these feelings are normal and they will pass.

I cannot tell you how long it will take you to recover emotionally, as everyone is different. In the long term, very few women ever forget their miscarriage and many women can recall with great clarity miscarriages that occurred twenty and thirty years previously. There are also particular times, the date when the baby would have been born, for instance, when you feel particularly sad. However, the initial sadness usually lessens over a few weeks or so, although it may be months before it fully resolves. If you feel that it is taking you a long time to recover, don't hesitate to go to your doctor.

If I wrote everything that I feel and know about how to cope with miscarriage, after two myself and what seems a lifetime of listening to the experiences of others, I would fill a book twice this size and still not do it justice. All I can do here is to give you some signposts. Talking to other parents who have been through the same experience can be immensely helpful, and there are two organisations which not only offer counselling, but which can also put you in touch with local support groups. The Miscarriage Association and SANDS (the Stillbirth and Neonatal Death Association) also have a number of leaflets and other information which you may find useful. For many years pregnancy loss was not something that was openly acknowledged. This attitude is changing and you will find the details of several recently published books in Appendix I.

Causes

The first thing you want to know is 'why'. The trouble with miscarriage is that symptoms often occur some time after the death of the baby. There is a tendency, therefore, to blame activities that take place immediately before, or at the time that symptoms occur, as being the cause of the miscarriage. And of course, because such activities were largely under your control, it becomes 'your fault'. Thus it is that I have heard hoovering, carrying heavy shopping, getting wet and cold, overwork, tiredness, riding a horse (or bicycle) and lovemaking put forward as a cause of a woman's miscarriage. What doesn't help either is Hollywood's depiction of miscarriage. Years of Hollywood weepies like *Gone with the Wind*, where heroines lost their babies with great clutchings of stomachs and groaning as a result of frights, falls and footloose men deserting them have, I am afraid, taken their toll, on our mothers' generation in particular. For the record, women have skied down mountains, competed in top class athletics and jumped out of planes (mostly it has to be said before they were aware that they were pregnant) without their babies coming to any harm. The only reason, incidentally, why horse riding is discouraged in pregnancy is because you might fall off and land heavily on your abdomen (which can be a cause of miscarriage); it is not because sitting with your legs apart or being jiggled about will cause you to lose your baby.

Although it is a gross generalisation, it remains the case that miscarriage in the first trimester is more likely to be because the baby has a problem, with later miscarriage being related to maternal or external factors. It is quite possible for a woman to have several miscarriages, each of which has a different cause.

Abut 60 per cent of early miscarriages are likely to be the

result of a non-recurring chromosome abnormality. You may, however, never know whether this was the cause of your miscarriage, because genetic testing is only possible in about 20 per cent of miscarriages because of lack of suitable material for testing (i.e. material that has not already died and in which it is clear which are maternal and which are fetal tissues).

I can't explain, I am afraid, *why* chromosome abnormalities occur – only embryo research is likely to reveal that – but I can explain a bit of the how. Each of the cells in the body has 23 pairs of chromosomes, except sperm and egg, which have 23 single chromosomes. If you think about it, were this not the case, when sperm and egg met up the fertilised egg would have 46 pairs of chromosomes, instead of 23. Instead of the normal sort of cell replication process, sperm and egg go through a curious process known as a reduction division (meiosis) in order to get to the 23 singles state. For men, this takes place in the testicles. For women, it takes place as the egg is travelling down the fallopian tube. Sometimes the reduction division isn't very efficient – one pair of chromosomes may fail to separate (a process called non-disjunction), so that the new gamete (egg or sperm) contains not 23 singles, but 22 singles and a pair. It also means that somewhere else there is a sperm or egg that just has 22 singles. The implications of this former process are that when sperm unites with egg, there will be 22 pairs, and a threesome or trisomy. The implication of the latter is that a fertilised egg will contain 22 pairs and a single (because the appropriate single is off hobnobbing elsewhere in a threesome).

A trisomy of chromosome 21 is the cause of Down's Syndrome and there are other trisomies, such as those causing Edwards or Patau Syndromes. Many trisomies are lethal to the baby. There are all sorts of other shenanigans that go on when chromosomes attempt to sort themselves out, and quite a high proportion of eggs and sperm are chromosomally abnormal as a result. This goes on in people who are perfectly normal and healthy in every other way and is part and parcel of the way we are. It is also the reason why, as a species, we are not very efficient about reproduction – there is a phenomenally high wastage rate of very early embryos – and this in part may explain why, despite everything else being right, there is only a 1 in 4 chance of pregnancy in any one cycle.

As women get older, their eggs are more likely to be chromosomally abnormal, since their eggs are the same age as they are, hence the increase in the incidence of abnormalities such as Down's Syndrome with age. Thus you can see that these sort of problems arise at conception. They are not caused by anything you did, or indeed didn't do. A final word before leaving chromosomes. Sometimes a fertilised egg may end up, as I have indicated, with 22 pairs and a threesome. The threesome might include two singles from the mother and a single from the father, or two singles from the father and one from the mother. These threesomes are a bit tricky to work with and cells don't much like them, so one of the threesome tends to get chucked out somewhere along the line – which might leave a proper pair, or alternatively a pair which both come from either the mother or the father. This phenomenon is called uniparental disomy and it would seem that it is associated with about 10 per cent of the type of miscarriage known as 'blighted ovum'.

Before telling you some further possible causes of miscarriage, it is worth saying that it is far easier to be positive about what didn't cause your miscarriage than about what did. You may feel that it is a heresy for me to say this, but in some ways searching for the cause of one-off miscarriage is an exercise in futility. For, having eliminated a range of possibilities, you are left with what? A nothing, a fuzzy mass of could-bes and maybes with which to torture yourself. There is a reason for your miscarriage, of course there is, but we are simply not clever enough yet to identify it; and even if we could identify it, it is more likely than not that we could do zip to prevent it happening again. Miscarriage is a tragedy, it wounds, it is something you will remember, clear as day, for the rest of your life. But it is part of life's rich pageant and has to be put firmly in that perspective.

SMOKING

Smoking almost doubles the risk of miscarriage. Other complications which are increased when the mother smokes are ectopic pregnancy, placenta praevia, placental abruption, premature labour. Every time the mother smokes an increased fetal heart rate is seen from 2 minutes and persists for 15 minutes following each smoking episode. Here is something that you can clearly do something about in a future pregnancy.

INFECTION

Viruses that are known to cause both malformation and miscarriage are rubella (prevention: check immunity before pregnancy, vaccinate if appropriate), cytomegalovirus (CMV) (prevention: usually picked up from infected children; handwashing and avoidance of contact with saliva sufficient), herpes (first attack in pregnancy only – prevention: condom use essential during pregnancy with new partner or if partner has genital herpes), parvovirus (prevention: avoid children with 'slapped cheek' rash) and toxoplasmosis (prevention: avoid emptying cat litter, garden with gloves, wash veg and salads before eating, avoid undercooked meat, unpasteurised goat's milk). It is not known whether it is the organism itself or the toxins liberated by the organism which causes the baby's death in these cases. It might be that fever generated by infections are the cause of miscarriage. Certainly if you have fever in pregnancy you should take prompt action to lower your temperature with medicines such as paracetamol which is widely regarded as being safe to take in pregnancy. If your occupation is that of farmer or shepherdess, there are special risks from bacterial infections associated with calving and lambing, and pregnant women should avoid involvement in these activities if they can. Syphilis is known to cause recurrent miscarriage but is easily diagnosed and treated, and is a rare cause of miscarriage in Britain. In general the infections I have mentioned will not cause recurrent miscarriage, because once a woman has been exposed to infection she is normally immune to reinfection. Minor coughs and colds are not harmful to pregnancy.

VDUS

I have put this as a category, only to scotch it. Repeated studies have shown that there is no increased risk of miscarriage associated with VDU usage.

TRAVEL

Air travel and long journeys are sometimes cited as causes of miscarriage. This is unlikely, but certainly if you are pregnant and are going on a long journey you should break frequently and walk about a bit when you do, as this restores a good bloodflow to the pelvic area.

UNCONTROLLED SYSTEMIC DISEASE

If you have an existing chronic disease that is not under good control, such as diabetes, systemic lupus, sickle cell anaemia, epilepsy or cardiovascular disease, you are more likely to have a miscarriage.

ABNORMALITIES OF THE REPRODUCTIVE TRACT

A miscarriage (usually at a later stage of pregnancy) may reveal an unexpected and previously unsuspected abnormality of the womb, such as an internal septate (division). Sometimes surgery is appropriate, although it may leave a scar which could affect future pregnancies. Here bed rest may have a value in helping to maintain subsequent pregnancies. There is a good chance that you will eventually have a healthy baby, although it may well be born prematurely. Fibroids are also a possible cause of miscarriage, although in general they have to be very large in order to disrupt a pregnancy. They can be surgically removed (a myomectomy), although this will leave an internal scar which in itself may cause problems (because it means that there are fewer places for an embryo to implant).

Cervical incompetence, in which the cervix is weaker than it should be, is a cause of second trimester miscarriage. It can be treated using a 'stitch', which is, just as it sounds, a piece of gynaecological embroidery work which circles the top of the cervix and is drawn tight to keep it shut. The stitch will be inserted in hospital, usually under general or epidural anaesthetic. A few days' rest in hospital will be necessary. The stitch is taken out at about 38 weeks and is easily removed, without the need for anaesthetic. There is a specific support group for women having this procedure (their address is in Appendix I). It is not likely to be the cause of a first trimester miscarriage.

IMMUNE FACTORS

Immune factors – the way in which the mother's defence system reacts to her baby – may be responsible for some blighted ovum and missed miscarriage types of miscarriage (see under·recurrent miscarriage, page 159, for a full explanation).

EXPOSURE TO TERATOGENS

A wide range of substances from radiation, to household chemicals, to alcohol, have the potential to cause miscarriage. Many women are concerned becuase they conceived in an alcoholic haze. The blastocyst (the ball of cells that becomes the embryo) is incredibly resistant to teratogens for the first two weeks (i.e. four weeks of pregnancy) and therefore it is possible to be reassuring on this point. And there have been one or two other babies conceived in similar circumstances. Here again, the knowledge that chemicals can cause miscarriage may not help one bit – you may worry whether breathing paint fumes when you were decorating, or having your hair permed, caused your miscarriage. If you start on this tack, you'll end up as a nervous wreck and almost certainly will not accurately identify the cause of your miscarriage.

NUTRITIONAL DEFICIENCIES

A similar point applies here, but see Chapter 4 on nutrition in pregnancy for further information.

ENDOMETRITIS

Another type of infection, this time of the womb lining by organisms such as ureaplasma or mycoplasma – both of which are commonly found in the vagina – which may cause miscarriage.

POLYCYSTIC OVARIAN DISEASE

Miscarriage is more common in women who have polycystic ovarian disease (in which the ovaries are studded with follicles). A finding common to women with polycystic ovaries is that they have high levels of luteinising hormone (LH). New types of treatment are being devised which can help prevent too much LH being secreted. This is, however, specialised treatment which you are unlikely to find outside of centres specialising in recurrent miscarriage. A simple blood test, or daily urine tests, will reveal whether this is the problem.

STRESS

Whilst there is a great deal of evidence to support the view that tender loving care gets more women with histories of miscarriage through pregnancy than any other 'treatment', and although this might lead one to think that the converse – i.e. stressful pregnancy – was a cause of miscarriage, there has never been any evidence to support this whatsoever. Worry about something else.

Molar pregnancies may masquerade as miscarriages, as indeed may ectopic pregnancies. Both are discussed in detail in other chapters.

Investigating Miscarriage

After one miscarriage investigation is unlikely and may indeed be futile in the vast majority of cases. You have a greater than 95 per cent chance of successful pregnancy next time around. Undertaking chromosome analysis of the fetal material is only possible in 20 per cent of cases, as indicated. In half of the cases investigated, no definite cause will be found. Even two miscarriages are much more likely to be a run of chromosomal bad luck than a specific problem. Having said all this, I personally believe that after two miscarriages you should ask for at least some testing. For instance, checking that your womb is normal and taking a blood sample to check antiphospholipid antibodies would be sensible. A full scale witch hunt for possible infection may not. In a recent publication, 'TORCH Screening Reassessed', the Public Health Laboratory Service recommended that testing for infections following a history of miscarriages should only be undertaken if there were symptoms, or alternatively if a woman had a definite history of contact (TORCH covers toxoplasma, rubella, cytomegalovirus and herpes), because the results are so inconclusive.

Recurrent Miscarriage

Recurrent miscarriage is defined as a history of three or more consecutive miscarriages. After three miscarriages, the chance that a specific problem is causing them becomes greater than the chance that they are simply random unrelated events. You should be aware that investigations can be extensive and still not reveal the cause, and that, as I said earlier, each miscarriage could have had a different cause.

CHROMOSOME ABNORMALITIES

A small proportion of recurrent miscarriages are the result of chromosome abnormalities in each parent, so-called balanced chromosome arrangements, which are not a cause of abnormality in the parent, but which may cause problems in the baby. There are a large number of different types of such chromosome anomalies and they require specialist interpretation by a clinical geneticist. About 4 per cent of recurrent miscarriages have this cause.

Some of the factors cited above, such as infection and problems with the size or shape of the womb, can be the cause of repeated miscarriage. Unsuspected thyroid disease can also be a cause.

SPERM ABNORMALITIES

Several cases have been reported of sperm abnormalities, specifically those in which there were more than usual numbers of double-headed sperm, being associated with repeated miscarriage. This caused the fertilised egg to have two sets of paternal chromosomes, and therefore to be miscarried at an early stage. Treatment involved separating abnormal sperm out of a sperm sample before using it to inseminate the woman.

IMMUNOLOGICAL PROBLEMS

It has been claimed that the majority of cases of repeated miscarriage have an immunological cause. Pregnancy is a complete contradiction, in that a foreign body is not only not challenged by the immune system, which is normally programmed to seek and destroy anything which is not 'self', but is allowed to prosper and grow inside the body. There is evidently some mechanism which allows the baby to 'hide' from the ever-vigilant immune system, although nobody has yet discovered what it is. Immune disorders of pregnancy takes one of three forms. In the first, antiphospholipid antibody syndrome, the mother's immune system turns against her own cells and tissues. This is also known as the lupus anticoagulant, or cardiolipin antibody. It can cause blood clots to form within the placenta and may be responsible for 10–20 per cent of recurrent miscarriages. Treatment is likely to involve one aspirin a day (aspirin thins the blood) in combination with prednisone (a steroid) or heparin (another blood thinner). The disease can easily be determined by the amounts of antiphospholipid antibody in a woman's bloodstream.

In women with the auto-immune disease lupus, a similar attack is mounted against the mother's body by her own immune system. In general, women would already be aware that they had lupus. Because it tends to flare up during pregnancy, and because it is associated with a higher than normal miscarriage rate, pregnant women with lupus need specialist care. St Thomas's Hospital in London specialises in this type of pregnancy.

Finally, the mother's body can reject the baby as if it were a foreign object. Because recurrent miscarriage appeared to be a disease of couples (i.e. if the woman changed her partner, the problem disappeared), a theory was proposed to explain this. It is said that, far from being very different, the parents were genetically very similar, particularly with regard to the genes that code for formation of the defence system (HLA genes), and because of this, whatever mechanism was responsible for protecting the baby wasn't being triggered as it should. A treatment, immunotherapy, was devised, which involved giving women injections of their husband's white blood cells before pregnancy occurred. The idea was that this sensitisation would be sufficient to 'switch off' the mother's immune system and therefore protect the pregnancy. I have vastly simplified something which is very complex indeed but this is the general gist of it.

An impressive trial of immunotherapy was published in 1985 by a group of doctors from St Mary's Hospital, London. Yet despite the excitement with which it was greeted, the success of the trial (70 per cent of women had pregnancies which went to term) and the continuing claims of the authors, they were never able to explain the immunological basis of their treatment. A number of other centres attempted to achieve similar results and none did. Gradually immuno-therapy fell out of favour, with intensive regimes of TLC being instituted in their place. It has to be said that, whichever of a great variety of treatments is used, pregnancy outcome is eventually successful in 70–90 per cent of cases.

Trying Again

Pregnancies that follow miscarriages are often difficult, in that no matter how perfectly the pregnancy seems to be proceed-ing, it is still beset with anxiety and ambivalence. You want to rejoice in it going well, but you somehow dare not do so. The experience of losing your baby may have made you feel so doubtful of success and afraid of further losses that you decide to put off having babies for quite a while. On the other hand, some parents feel that they want to try again immediately. This is understandable, but may not be the best course of action in the long run, because they may not have allowed themselves enough time to grieve for the previous baby.

Doctors differ considerably in their advice to couples

wanting to try again after a miscarriage. Your body will certainly need more time to recover from a later miscarriage – at least three months – than from an early one. If you have had an early miscarriage, it is wise to wait until you have had at least one normal period, simply because otherwise it will be difficult to date your next pregnancy accurately. In truth, there is no set answer. It is down to how you feel about another pregnancy and when you feel ready to try again.

A natural reaction, once you do conceive again, is to keep the news of your pregnancy a secret. In some ways this can backfire. You need all the support you can get through the early months of another pregnancy, and not telling anyone deprives you of that support. Enlist the help of your GP at a very early stage and ask him or her to refer you for an early scan as this will help reassure you that the pregnancy is normal. Most GPs are sympathetic and aware of the special anxieties that women who have had miscarriages face.

Getting in the best possible shape, both physically and emotionally, in preparation for the next pregnancy is a very positive step to take and will make you feel that you have done everything possible for a healthy pregnancy. You should certainly stop smoking, keep alcohol intake to a minumum, try to eat as healthily as possible as well as getting fit. But leading a saintly life is no guarantee that you will not have another miscarriage. Whatever we might believe, we cannot manage our pregnancies in the way that some would suggest we can. Chromosome abnormalities, which cause the majority of miscarriages, are chance events that we cannot control and, rather like tossing a coin ten times and getting ten heads or ten tails in a row, it is possible that it will happen again, but unlikely.

I have kept back the best news, so that they are the last thing you read in this chapter: statistics. After one miscarriage you have a greater than 95 per cent chance of a full term pregnancy next time around. Even after two miscarriages, your chances only drop to 80 per cent or so, and after three there is still a 70 per cent chance of successful pregnancy. Thus the odds of you having a baby after a miscarriage are very heavily stacked in your favour. Grieve for the baby you have lost, but never think that parenthood is something you will be denied.

9

Ectopic Pregnancy

If you are reading this chapter, you may well have already had an ectopic pregnancy – i.e. in which a fertilised egg embedded itself somewhere other than in your womb. You may have been completely unprepared for the diagnosis, especially if pregnancy wasn't on your agenda. Even if you were planning pregnancy, the varied symptoms caused by an ectopic may have misled you and your doctors. Either way, a medical emergency may have ensued, leaving you feeling particularly vulnerable and concerned for the future. You may then have turned to pregnancy guides for further information and found nothing, giving you to suppose that the dramatic situation you went through was very rare. Not so.

In truth, the number of ectopic pregnancies has reached epidemic proportions. In America, ectopic pregnancies have tripled in number over the last twenty years. Here in Britain, the figures are less dramatic but are still increasing year by year. In the States about 1 in every 60 pregnancies is ectopic, whilst the figures in Britain are about 1 in every 200 pregnancies. Partly because deaths from other causes have fallen, ectopic pregnancy has become the major cause of maternal mortality in the first trimester of pregnancy, accounting for some 10 per cent of all maternal deaths.

It is not, however, a situation of unrelenting gloom. With the advent of transvaginal ultrasound, it is possible to diagnose 90 per cent of cases correctly, before life-threatening haemorrhage occurs.

But before detailing the causes, symptoms and consequences of ectopic pregnancy, I must tell you about the
fallopian tubes, because they are the villains of this piece.
Unlikely though it sounds, I am always reminded of them
when I go to Heathrow on the tube. As you come out of the
underground, there is a long corridor with two moving
walkways, one going into the airport and the other leaving it.
If you heave your suitcase on to the walkway, it obligingly
carries it for you, dumping it rather unceremoniously at the
other end. Just like that corridor at Heathrow, the fallopian
tube is a two-way transport system. It carries, not people and
luggage, but sperm and eggs and its moving walkways are
powered by the concerted beating of tiny little hairs called cilia
which line parts of the tube. Once the cilia beating stops, for
whatever reason – perhaps there is a gap where there aren't any
cilia, for instance – whatever is being transported will come to
a grinding halt, as your suitcase would if Heathrow had a
power cut. Transport within the tube is also affected by the
contractions of its muscular wall, which moves the contents
along rather in the same way that food is made to move
through the gut. If you think about it, the tube is doing a
pretty unique transport job – after all, at the same time that
sperm want to go up, the egg is wanting to go down. The
fallopian tube normally manages to satisfy both parties, moving
them in opposite directions almost simultaneously.

There are several distinct areas to the tube (see diagram).
The fimbriated end (fimbria means fringe) serves to pick up
the egg, in an exercise which is rather like one of those cup
and ball games. The start of the tube, the ampulla, is not as
muscular as the remainder of the tube but contains lots of cilia.
The main section of the tube is narrow, muscular and
increasingly less ciliated as it moves towards its junction with
the womb. About 85 per cent of ectopics occur in the

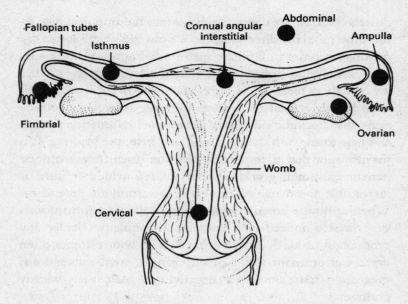

Diagram showing different sites of ectopic pregnancy.

ampullary section of the tube and 5 per cent in the long straight bit (isthmus). In general, the nearer to the junction with the womb, the more severe the problems are likely to be. Other sites of implantation are the cervix, ovary and the abdomen.

The directional movements in the fallopian tubes vary during the menstrual cycle and are influenced by two pacemakers, one in the ampulla and the other in the isthmus. They are the body's equivalent of the burly chaps beating drums to dictate oar speed in Roman galleys, and can send different signals to the portion of the tube above or below them. During your period, the net flow is directed towards your womb, in an effort to prevent menstrual blood refluxing into the tubes. Just before you ovulate, the force is outwards in order to pick up the egg and move it into the ampullar area. At the same time, the directional force from the womb is just the opposite in order to facilitate sperm moving towards the egg. The general plot is that by the time the fertilised egg reaches the womb, a week or so after having been fertilised, it will have already started to develop the little finger-like projections, the chorionic villi, that will start the implantation process and help form, with the womb lining's help, the placenta. It is the placenta that is responsible for the pregnancy hormone human chorionic gonadotrophin (hCG), which in turn is responsible for many of the early symptoms of pregnancy. When a tubular pregnancy occurs this placental formation is very limited indeed and there is consequently hardly any production of hCG. This is why women with ectopics often don't feel pregnant and, not surprisingly, why conventional pregnancy tests are often negative or only very weakly positive.

The womb is a great big tough organ, capable of being distended. The fallopian tube is not. There are three possible things that can happen to a tubal pregnancy and these depend to some extent on its location and the stage of pregnancy. If the embryo dies, spontaneous regression often occurs, with the embryo being resorbed. This is probably a very common event indeed, with a woman never knowing that she has even been pregnant, much less had an ectopic.

The second scenario is one in which the pregnancy aborts, because the placenta separates from the wall of the tube, and the embryo is expelled into the abdominal cavity via the fimbriated end of the tube. Unless one of the blood vessels in the tube is injured in the process, bleeding usually stops quite quickly. Again, a woman may not be aware of this. Bleeding may continue, however, until complete separation takes place. The female body has the equivalent of a sump – it's called the pouch of Douglas and it's a blind cul-de-sac behind the womb. You can use a needle attached to a syringe, passing it through the vaginal wall, to suck out its contents – a technique called culdocentesis. If the pouch contains fluid or blood cells, it's a bit of a giveaway, especially if, on an ultrasound scan, the womb is empty and a pregnancy test is positive. No further action, apart from careful observation, is required and recovery is usually quick. The final scenario is a complete rupture of the tube, which may involve catastrophic internal bleeding and shock.

Symptoms

If you had to go in for a gynaecological masterclass and were asked for the classic symptoms of ectopic pregnancy, you would dutifully write down: pain, vaginal bleeding and amenorrhoea (no periods). However, as ever, real life tends to ignore what is written in the medical textbooks. The bewildering manifestations of ectopic pregnancy can confuse even the most experienced of gynaecologists, and as a result there is no gynaecologist who can put his hand on his heart and honestly say that he has never misdiagnosed an ectopic. Add to this the fact that you may not even believe pregnancy to have been possible (because you were using contraception effectively, you thought, or because you had recently had what seemed like a normal period) and the possibilities for a delay in correct diagnosis are legion. About 25 per cent of ectopics are incorrectly diagnosed initially. The better news is that about twice as many ectopic pregnancies are suspected as actually occur, which is indicative of the higher index of suspicion these days. The most common conditions which can be confused with ectopic pregnancy are ovarian problems (e.g.

torsion or rupture of cysts), other pregnancy problems (threatened miscarriage), pelvic inflammatory disease, acute appendicitis and other gut problems, and kidney disease.

About 90 per cent of women with ectopics have abdominal pain, usually in the lower abdomen. Often it starts as a dull, nagging pain caused by the stretching of the tube, which may also be crampy, coming and going rather like period pain. The pain may then get sharper. It may be more intense to one side and the abdomen will be tender to the touch, especially around the navel. A mass may be felt, sometimes on the other side of the ectopic. On internal examination, any touch to the cervix will cause pain. In general, pain precedes any bleeding and it may increase if the tube ruptures, and then either lessen considerably or continue to be severe as the loss of blood begins to irritate the lining of the abdomen. Often women report shoulder pain, which is due to the diaphragm being irritated by blood in the abdominal cavity. If there is internal bleeding, there may be sudden giddiness, fainting, nausea and other symptoms of shock.

About 70 per cent of women with ectopics will report either being late with their period or, more confusingly, having had a period but its having been irregular − usually lighter than normal. About 15 per cent of women will have had no alteration to their normal periods.

In about half of all cases of ectopic pregnancy, there is either mild or intermittent dark red or brown discharge/bleeding. This occurs because the levels of pregnancy hormones are so low that they are insufficient to prevent shedding of the womb lining.

Diagnosis

Conventional pregnancy testing (using urine) and simple examination of the abdomen are not effective in predicting either the presence or absence of an ectopic pregnancy. Fortunately, with the advent of more advanced ultrasound scanning and blood tests for pregnancy, more ectopic pregnancies are being recognised before the tube has ruptured and tubal loss is inevitable.

The first step is a pregnancy test on urine. If that is positive, ultrasound scanning is indicated. If the test is negative, the test should be repeated on blood. The test used is called beta hCG. The so-called 'beta chain' of hCG is what makes it different from another reproductive hormone, luteinising hormone. The beta hCG tests are very sensitive indeed, as they need to be, because hCG levels are so low in ectopic pregnancies. If the test is positive, then once again ultrasound is indicated. If the womb is shown to be empty, then another blood test for beta hCG will be undertaken, this time to measure the exact quantity present. There is a so-called discriminatory zone which is a level of beta hCG at which a sac should be seen in the womb. If it is not seen, then the likelihood of an ectopic is greater than 90 per cent. Above this level, the next course would be laparoscopy. If below this level, another hCG test would be undertaken forty-eight hours later. If the level of hCG has risen by more than two-thirds, normal pregnancy is highly likely (hCG levels rise in a set pattern in early pregnancy). If it is lower, then the scan should be repeated. Frequently these days, hospitals have access to vaginal ultrasonography, which has revolutionised the diagnosis of ectopics, as they can indicate the presence of the baby in the womb as early as 5 weeks of pregnancy (i.e. just three weeks after conception). It is possible, of course, to have one pregnancy in the womb and one in a tube, but this is rare in the extreme (1 in 30,000). There are certain pregnancies, for instance those following tubal surgery, where it should be assumed that pregnancy is ectopic until proved otherwise. The fact that vaginal ultrasonography can be so positive in its diagnosis so early in pregnancy is a source of considerable comfort to these women.

Finally, one less serious note. Accident and emergency departments are much more alert to the possibility of ectopic pregnancy these days and the general rule is to assume any woman is pregnant until proven otherwise. Sometimes an over-cautious houseman will insist (as he probably should) that he run a pregnancy test even though you may have assured him of your celibacy, and that if you were pregnant it would rival the Virgin Mary in the miracle stakes. A woman later found to have appendicitis told me that she had arrived in casualty with her husband who had just come home the week before after six months abroad. He was not amused about the pregnancy testing. However, should you ever be in this situation, for the record, a negative beta hCG virtually excludes an ectopic, or indeed any other sort of pregnancy.

One other hormone test may be used. Blood progesterone levels which are greater than a certain amount virtually assure a normal pregnancy. However, progesterone tests take twenty-four hours to produce results and they are only of use in those women who are pregnant following spontaneous ovulation (i.e. not those pregnant following fertility treatment) which is why they are now used only very rarely. In fact, as vaginal ultrasonography becomes more widely available, it is likely that blood tests will become less and less important in clinical practice in the diagnosis of ectopic pregnancy.

Treatment

Traditionally the treatment for ectopic pregnancy has been to remove the affected tube. Today the treatment is much more conservative, with every effort being made to preserve the tube if at all possible, and this strategy has been aided by the earlier stage at which ectopics are now diagnosed. It used to be believed that conserving the tube in which an ectopic had occurred would merely make it more likely that an ectopic would happen again. In fact, reviewing conservative surgery over a twenty-year period, it was shown that in those with a second ectopic pregnancy the ectopic occurred just as often in the previously uninvolved tube.

In general, if the ectopic has been finally diagnosed using a laparoscope, under general anaesthetic, a procedure called a laparotomy will follow straight on, without you regaining consciousness. This will involve making an incision, about 2 cm across, just above your pubic hairline. However, if the tube has not ruptured, this may not be necessary. If the tube is intact, the pregnancy may be shelled out through a small incision in the tubal wall made by a laser. There is no bleeding (the blood vessels are sealed as they are cut) and the incision in the tube heals up by itself (a salpingostomy). If the incision is stitched up, it is called a salpingotomy. Occasionally it may be necessary to remove a small section of the tube, and the two free ends then rejoined.

Another newer method is to inject a powerful anti-cancer drug directly into the ectopic. This will stop it growing, and it is reabsorbed by the body leaving the tube intact. The drug is called methotrexate, and this technique is still the subject of trials. An alternative method of administration of this drug is intravenously on alternate days for seven days. It is only suitable if there is no bleeding and for ectopics of very early gestation.

As I have indicated, the name of the game these days is conservation and everything possible will be done to keep your tube intact. Luckily for you, if your ectopic is discovered in an unruptured state you have the time to discuss the surgery and what it entails with your gynaecologist beforehand. Don't be a shrinking violet; assume nothing and demand the fullest possible information about what is going to happen and what your future prospects are. One tip, however, culled from years of dealing with gynaecologists – try not to be aggressive. Gynaecologists are actually great team players; never forget that you are potentially the team star. They want to make it work for you, because if it works for you, it works for them too.

If the tube has ruptured, it has to be removed (salpingectomy), and this is emergency surgery. Rarely, if the ectopic has involved the ovary or the blood supply to it, the ovary will have to be removed as well. Surgeons do not do this unless they absolutely have to. However, your life is their first consideration.

There is a third treatment strategy which is basically 'wait and see' – the ironically and wholly inappropriately named 'expectant management'. You are hospitalised, and serial beta hCG testing is undertaken whilst your vital signs are constantly monitored. This might sound a rather alarming way of doing things, but in truth many ectopic pregnancies probably do not rupture dramatically but will slowly undergo resorption. In fact, early detection of ectopics that would normally have resolved by themselves may account for some of the increase in ectopic numbers.

Coping

If your ectopic was in the very early weeks of pregnancy and you had a laparotomy, you may have only been an out-patient, or at the most stayed in hospital a day or so. If the tube ruptured, you will probably have stayed in hospital up to a week, or perhaps more, depending on your state when you came into hospital, how much blood you lost, etc. If this was what happened to you, with its subsequent haemorrhage and high medical drama, you may have been completely out of it and not aware of the gravity of your situation. In fact, having had surgery, you may feel a great deal better than you did before. Your partner, on the other hand, will have been through the mill.

An ectopic pregnancy is still a pregnancy. You still lost a baby. Because you may have been so very ill, the sorrow you feel about losing the baby may take a back seat in other people's minds in comparison to concerns about your immediate health. It may be especially difficult for your partner, who perhaps saw you when your life was on the line, to appreciate what you feel about losing the baby. He's just glad to have you in one piece. Although people will tell you how ill you were, or how near you came to the tube rupturing, it may not sink in for some time. When it does you may feel very wobbly. You may also feel very concerned about prospects for future pregnancy, not just because of possible infertility, but because in your case pregnancy was a potentially life-threatening condition. It is very difficult to contemplate pregnancy again, even if the odds are stacked in your favour (the exact odds are discussed later), when you think that you may be putting your life in jeopardy. This may affect your partner more than you and may possibly affect your lovemaking for a while, if he associates conception with life-and-death drama in a hospital casualty department.

If your ectopic pregnancy ended up as an emergency admission to hospital, you will have discovered that there is no privacy with an ectopic. Everyone knows that you were pregnant, which you may not have wanted. Sometimes an ectopic is a very unwelcome way of discovering that you were pregnant. Psychologically you may feel very rattled by this experience, not having had time to assimilate the fact that you were pregnant, let alone come to terms with losing the baby. Another difficulty is that when you try again, it will be against a background of people being very anxious on your behalf, if not actually hostile – 'How could you think of putting yourself through it again?'

In general, ectopic pregnancy cases are admitted to gynaecology wards. This may add to your feeling of being a medical case, rather than a mother who is losing her baby. However, it is true to say that staff on gynaecology wards have more time to talk than in the frantically busy antenatal wards, where almost everyone else will be pregnant and a constant reminder of the baby you have either lost or are about to lose.

If a gynaecologist reached you before your tube ruptured, and you had subsequent surgery to remove the ectopic, you may wonder whether, if not for this action, your baby would have continued to grow and whether you did the right thing in agreeing to have the pregnancy removed. As I have explained, the dangers of tubal abruption are to some extent dependent on the location of the ectopic. Those nearest the womb, in so-called interstitial sites, rupture with often catastrophic haemorrhage and haemorrhage is the cause of death in nearly 90 per cent of ectopic-related maternal deaths. To leave a pregnancy in this site is culpably to dice with death. For pregnancies in this and other tubal sites, death is a certainty for the baby, which cannot develop properly. As for abdominal pregnancy, up to 25 per cent will reach viability, but for these survivors the risk of deformity is very high, with almost half the babies having joint deformities, facial asymmetry, etc., mostly caused by the lack of the normal surrounding pond of fluid.

Different people take different times to recover from a physical trauma like this. You should be mousy quiet for at least a week after your release from hospital, and thereafter you shouldn't be toting barges or lifting bales for at least a month. Driving shouldn't be on the agenda either, because sudden braking can strain the abdomen. You may continue to have some bleeding for a bit and you should use pads not tampons, because of the risk of infection. When your period returns, it's fine to go back to tampons. Your first period may be quite painful. Getting back to making love may take time. Orgasms, even if stimulated manually, may be a bit painful for a few weeks but it is an important time to be close. Even though it might have been a very early pregnancy loss, and the advice would normally be to wait until the return of a normal period before trying again, you may want to leave it a bit longer than this.

Causes

There is a considerable geographic variation to ectopic pregnancy. In Jamaica, there is an ectopic rate of 1 in 25 births. Women over 35 years old, non-whites, or those with a history of infertility are at the greatest risk.

PREVIOUS TUBAL INFECTIONS OR SURGERY

Previous pelvic infections caused by certain sexually transmitted diseases, such as chlamydia and gonorrhea, or endometritis (infection in the lining of the womb) following the birth of a previous baby can all predispose to a tubal infection. Such infections cause damage to the inside of the fallopian tube, causing straps of tissue to grow across the tube which interfere with the transport of the fertilised egg to the womb. These infections may also damage the little cilia that would normally be such an effective transport system. As I explained, if there is a gap in the cilia, the egg may come to a complete halt.

PREVIOUS ABDOMINAL OR TUBAL SURGERY

If you have had previous pelvic or abdominal surgery, and if blood got into the fallopian tubes during it, tubal adhesions may result from the irritation of the inside surface of the tube. Previous tubal surgery is probably the greatest risk factor of all and if you get pregnant following tubal surgery, you should assume that you have an ectopic pregnancy until proved otherwise.

IVF TREATMENT

There is an increased risk of an ectopic with in vitro fertilisation (IVF). There is a strange irony in this, because IVF is the method of choice for those with blocked fallopian tubes. You might think that because the tubes are bypassed, ectopics should be unlikely. Unfortunately, perhaps because of the damage that necessitated the IVF in the first place, ectopic pregnancy is a risk with both IVF and gamete intra-fallopian transport (GIFT). In addition, there is a 3 per cent increased incidence of ectopics associated with the type of ovulation-inducing drugs, such as clomiphene citrate (Clomid) and human menopausal gonadotrophin (Pergonal), often used in conjunction with IVF. If you go back to the section on the working of the tube, you will remember that the cilia and their drum beaters were able to alter the direction and strength of beat at different stages of the menstrual cycle. The signals for 'all to the right, boys' or 'eyes down and to the left' are the different levels and ratios of oestrogen and progesterone at the different stages of the cycle. Having said this, it is perhaps not surprising that drugs which alter this balance affect tubal transport. It is also thought, on the same tack, that some hormonal imbalances affect the tubes. For instance, a low progesterone level can cause weak propulsive force in the tube.

CONTRACEPTIVE USE

As a working rule, between 1 in 20 to 1 in 30 IUD (coil)-associated pregnancies are ectopic, compared with about 1 in 200 pregnancies amongst non-IUD users. There is confusion as to why this should be so. The coil is very effective at preventing normal pregnancy but not so good at preventing ectopic pregnancies, therefore the rate of ectopics amongst IUD users will seem to be high, because there are comparatively fewer normal pregnancies associated with IUD use. To some extent this is statistical doublespeak. A more convincing explanation is that there may be IUD-related inflammation in the tubes of IUD users. This is borne out by the fact that studies relate frequency of ectopics to duration of use of IUDs; histological studies indicate the presence of inflammatory cells present in the tubes of IUD users even though they may have no symptoms of infection; and finally by the fact that pelvic infections, especially by chlamydia, are notoriously silent. The sort of IUDs that are progestogen-loaded are particularly linked to ectopics.

It has been said that using the 'mini-pill', which contains progestogen without oestrogen, predisposes women to ectopic pregnancy. The evidence for this is weak. There are several theories but the most likely is that the progestogens modify tubal function in some way.

An ectopic is ten times more likely if 'morning after' contraception fails, once again because of its high oestrogen level. Up to a third of pregnancies in women in whom sterilisation has failed will be ectopic, depending on the method used for sterilisation.

SMOKING

Maternal smoking at time of conception is known to be associated with an increased risk of ectopic. Passive smoking is not associated with increased risk.

ENDOMETRIOSIS

The presence of endometrial tissue outside the womb apparently increases the receptivity of the fertilised egg to an ectopic implantation. There may also be a physical effect in that the tubes may become distorted or kinked by external adhesions, creating internal pockets in which the fertilised egg may linger too long.

ABNORMALITIES IN THE EGG

Here we enter the realm of theory. Intrinsic abnormalities of the fertilised egg could be responsible for ectopic pregnancy. It is also possible that the egg migrates from one ovary to the tube on the opposite side via an extrauterine or an intrauterine route – so-called transmigration. Potentially this may delay the fertilised egg's transport to the womb. Accordingly those little chorionic fingers I spoke of earlier may be present before the egg reaches the safety of the womb cavity and will implant themselves in the fallopian tube.

You may have read through the preceding list of causes to find that, save for the last, which is anybody's guess, you have none of the above risk factors. In fact, when people ask me about ectopic pregnancy, and I dutifully run through the causes, nine times out of ten I know she will wail that none of them applies to her. The next question is almost invariably a variation on 'Was it something I did?' The answer is very simple. No. Life is quite guilt-inducing enough without blaming yourself for something that is patently *not* your fault. Grieve for the baby you lost, accept that you had an ectopic, but for heaven's sake don't torture yourself that you caused it. You didn't.

Trying Again

You may feel devastated by an ectopic pregnancy and feel very unsure about another pregnancy. There is, however, good reason to be hopeful. Firstly, nine out of ten women will conceive a normal pregnancy next time around, there being a recurrence rate of about 10 per cent. For those with an infertility problem, the recurrence rate is higher – 15 per cent – but this still means the odds are heavily stacked in favour of normal pregnancy. For those with previous tubal surgery, even if that tubal surgery was sterilisation, I am afraid it is a case of assuming that the pregnancy will be tubal until proved otherwise.

The next piece of positive news is that these days, especially if you have had a previous ectopic, very early scanning using vaginal ultrasound is available. This will reassure you right from the start that the pregnancy is normal, or at very worst tell you at the earliest possible stage that you have an ectopic, thereby giving the best chance of non-damaging forms of resolution.

If you have lost a tube, you may be very concerned about future pregnancy. It used to be assumed that your chances of pregnancy would be reduced, not because you were intrinsically less fertile, but because eggs are released from alternate ovaries and therefore it was assumed that you only had half the chances of conceiving of someone with two tubes. This is probably not true, as the egg can migrate to the other tube.

Sometimes conception seems to take for ever and it may be worth having an investigation with something called falloposcopy. This uses a new fibre-optic endoscope, with an outside diameter of just 0.5 mm, to look inside your tubes. The falloposcope is inserted via the cervix and no surgical incisions or anaesthetics are required. It is not yet widely available and is still being evaluated. From preliminary work it would seem that appearances can be deceiving. Sometimes the outside of your tubes may look fine but the inside be a mess, or equally, the outside look dreadful, but the inside be a gynaecologist's dream. Adhesions may have formed following the ectopic and it may be possible to resolve these laparoscopically.

What you do if you discover your tubes are a mess depends to some extent on your age. If you are younger, tubal surgery may do the trick. If you are older, you may feel that you don't have the time to wait and see whether the tubal surgery has worked, and may want to bypass this procedure, depending on what chances of success your gynaecologist gives you, and go straight for IVF. Once again, there is good news in that IVF was designed precisely for people like you with damaged tubes and it is for you that IVF holds the greatest chances of successful pregnancy. Don't be daunted. Go for it.

Summary

Ectopic pregnancy can be a life-threatening condition, and is the single largest cause of maternal mortality in the first three months of pregnancy. The numbers of ectopics have increased dramatically over the last twenty years, and although the increasing incidence of sexually transmitted disease and consequent tubal damage may be much to blame, it is apparent that the cause of an ectopic pregnancy may still be a mystery which only future embryo research may be able to solve. However, thanks to vaginal ultrasonography, more ectopics are being diagnosed before tubal rupture occurs, giving the greatest possible chance of pregnancy thereafter.

10

Molar Pregnancy

About one in every two thousand pregnancies is a so-called 'molar' pregnancy. To begin with, a woman may have every reason to believe that she is expecting a baby. She will have missed one period or more, the pregnancy test will have been very strongly positive, and she may be experiencing all the classic signs of pregnancy. She may even feel that she's a bit bigger than she would expect for her dates. In addition she may be having particularly bad morning sickness. Frequently, however, such a woman will find that she has a bit of vaginal bleeding, often brownish in colour, and may think that she is having a miscarriage.

However, when the woman is examined no fetal heartbeat can be heard and no heartbeat or indeed any fetal parts can be seen on scan. The scan may just have a white 'snowstorm' appearance. A blood test may reveal exceptional levels of the pregnancy hormone, human chorionic gonadotrophin (hCG), and the woman will be told that she has a hydatidiform (pronounced hyda-tidi-form) mole.

Mole in this context has nothing to do with a mole on your skin, nor a garden mole, it just means a mass. 'Hydatid' is a clear, fluid-filled cyst and taken together the term refers to a mass consisting of fluid-filled cysts — think of something looking like a bunch of fluid-filled grapes. The reason why hydatidiform mole is of special concern is because, depending on the type of mole, there is a risk of developing a type of cancer known as a gestational trophoblastic tumour (GTT). It used to be that these types of cancer had a very poor outlook indeed. Today, thanks to intensive medical research and diligent monitoring, this situation has been transformed, with an almost 100 per cent cure rate for the most frequently encountered type of mole.

Causes

Why does a mole develop and what on earth does trophoblastic mean? To answer both questions, I need to take you back to the very earliest stages of pregnancy. Soon after conception, rapid division of the fertilised egg takes place, so that very soon a ball of cells is formed. The outer layer of these cells is called the trophoblast and is initially responsible for the early nutrition of the embryo, but its principle job is to form the placenta. It rapidly forms, with other cells, into a sort of double envelope which surrounds the inner cluster of cells which is to become the embryo. The outer layer of this envelope is called the chorion. Bits of the trophoblast chorion sandwich are then pushed out, forming little finger-like projections of cells called chorionic villi. At this stage, the embryo looks a bit like a sputnik. Once in contact with the wall of the womb, these little fingers of trophoblast, by enzyme action, burrow into the womb's muscular wall, thus gaining an anchorage point and forming the placenta. Of course, only some of the projections on the 'sputnik', those in contact with the womb wall, will develop into the placenta. All the others, which point into the uterine cavity, will gradually waste away.

Trophoblast is potentially very invasive stuff, and from one point of view this is good because it favours as large a development of placental tissue as possible. However, how does it know when to stop doing its invasive bit? A mole is formed when part or all of the trophoblast gets out of control and undergoes degenerative changes. Sometimes, for reasons we'll go into later, no fetal development is possible and the conception remains as an undifferentiated ball of cells. Sometimes there is enough proper placental tissue to nourish an embryo through its very early stage, but almost invariably the embryo fails to develop properly, dies, and is soon resorbed. Depending on how much of the trophoblast is involved, the mole is classified either as complete or partial. In a complete mole, there never was a baby. In a partial mole there was a baby at the very beginning, although almost invariably there will be no baby by the time the mole is diagnosed. Although this sounds fairly clearcut, in practice distinguishing between the two is not always easy and detailed pathological investigation is required to determine the status of the mole. The majority of molar pregnancies are complete moles, with about 20 per cent being partial moles. But how do they happen?

You will remember that in every cell in your body you have 23 pairs of chromosomes, the microscopic structures that are repositories for the instruction manuals that are your genes. There is one exception to this rule. In sperm and egg, there are not 23 pairs, but 23 single chromosomes, so that when sperm and egg join up, there are once again 23 pairs of chromosomes. Part of the sperm manufacturing process that goes on in the testicle includes the so-called reduction division (meiosis) that ensures a chromosomal half measure in each sperm. However, in women, the reduction division occurs not in the ovary, but as the egg is moving down the fallopian tube. The half set of chromosomes that are excess to requirements are packaged up in something called a polar body which is pushed out of the egg whilst it is still on the move. Sometimes the packing up and pushing out is a bit over-enthusiastic, and as a consequence some eggs have no genetic material in them at all. Thus it is that a sperm can fertilise an empty egg. The resultant ball of cells will have a 46XX chromosome pattern, because subsequent cell division just leads to duplication of the sperm's genetic material. This material contains sufficient information to allow for the growth of the placenta (and it is the placenta, formed by trophoblast, that manufactures hCG, hence the positive pregnancy test), but there is not enough genetic material for a baby to be formed. Occasionally the chromosome pattern may be 46XY, because two sperm have fertilised an empty egg. Both these scenarios result in a complete hydatidiform mole.

The plot that results in a partial hydatidiform mole is a little different. Two sperm fertilise an apparently normal egg, resulting in a chromosome pattern which is triploid (three elements), one being maternal in origin and two paternal, either 69XXY, 69XXX or 69XYY. Here a baby can be formed, but because of the chromosome configuration it will have multiple congenital anomalies and will quickly die. Triploid chromosome patterns are not that uncommon, and by no means all of them result in molar pregnancy; they are a common finding following miscarriage.

It is possible for there to be a normal baby in association with a mole, if the pregnancy is a non-identical twin one, in which only one of the sacs is affected by molar changes. This is rare.

The common strand in both complete and partial mole is a double complement of paternal chromosomes. This is clearly abnormal, so it can be seen that a molar pregnancy is dictated right from the moment of conception and is not caused or influenced by any other factor that occurred between conception and diagnosis.

There are several theories as to why this should happen. A

defect in the egg is a possibility, and this theory is strengthened by the fact that molar pregnancy is a progressive risk with age, a woman of 50 having a 400 times greater chance of having one than a woman of 25. It is also more common in teenage pregnancy.

There are many striking features connected to the incidence of molar pregnancy across the world which may give some clues as to its cause. The incidence is about 1 in 2,000 in Britain, but in Asian countries this may rise to 1 in 200 pregnancies. It is now thought that this difference may have been exaggerated by different diagnostic practices, especially since immigrant Filipino women in America are known to have a similar incidence to the rest of the American population. But molar pregnancy is only half as frequent in black women, leading to the conclusion that there is a genetic element as well, perhaps, as an environmental element. Since you can do nothing about your race, or your age, or the country you live in, it follows that there is nothing you can do to prevent having another molar pregnancy. Actually the risks of having another are very slight – just 2 per cent – so the odds are heavily stacked in favour of normal pregnancy.

Symptoms

Symptoms for complete and partial mole are the same, although a partial mole may not show the symptoms as often. The most common 'alerting' symptom is bleeding from the womb, which is usually not profuse and which is often brownish. The womb may be bigger than might be expected (or sometimes smaller with a partial mole). There may be abdominal pain because the abnormal levels of hCG have caused cysts to form temporarily in the ovaries. Sickness is a very common complaint, with 25 per cent of women having the type of excessive nausea and vomiting called hyperemesis. About half of women will pass some of the grapelike vesicles present in the womb through the vagina. For reasons which are not clear, 30 per cent of women with a molar pregnancy will develop pre-eclampsia (see Chapter 11) before 24 weeks of pregnancy. A small number of women may develop signs of their thyroid having been affected, with symptoms such as sweating, increased heart rate, intolerance to heat, etc.

Diagnosis

Ultrasound is the most valuable tool for diagnosing the presence of a mole, resulting in a very characteristic pattern of multiple diffuse echoes, almost as if you had a black and white television on the blink. In a normal pregnancy, hCG levels gradually increase until around day 70–100 of pregnancy and then drop sharply. In a molar pregnancy, hCG levels are persistently high, or, earlier in pregnancy, are much higher than might be expected, particularly with complete mole. Partial mole levels of hCG in early pregnancy may be more or less normal.

Sometimes symptoms of molar pregnancy prompt diagnostic procedures. But it is sometimes the case that a woman thinks she is having a miscarriage, usually of the missed abortion type (see Chapter 8) and only after she has had a D & C is she told that it was a molar pregnancy.

Treatment

Once the mole has been diagnosed, immediate surgery to remove it from the womb is indicated. Under general anaesthetic, the womb is very carefully evacuated, using a suction technique, and the inside of the womb scraped hard (curettage). Because trophoblast is so well supplied with blood vessels, haemorrhage is always a risk and access to appropriate transfusion services is essential. With specialist services, however, evacuating a mole is nearly always accomplished without problems.

Follow-Up

In the vast majority of cases molar pregnancy has no more immediate consequences than any other failed pregnancy. Nevertheless you may feel devastated by it, partly perhaps because you may have felt so ill beforehand, but also because of concerns about future pregnancies and indeed concern for yourself. Nobody can even pronounce 'hydatidiform'; very few people have heard of the condition, let alone written about it for the layman, and it's all too easy for you and your partner and family to hear the word 'cancer' and just shut off, hearing nothing further. Stop right there; this is not a horror story.

There are two types of cancer that can develop following a molar pregnancy: choriocarcinoma and invasive mole (actually this latter isn't a true cancer). The risk of a choriocarcinoma after a complete mole is not more than 3 per cent; that of invasive mole about 10 per cent. Only 5 per cent of women who have had a complete mole pregnancy will require treatment. It is a very treatable type of cancer (with a virtually 100 per cent cure rate if detected before it spreads out of the womb), but this excellent prognosis depends on meticulous follow-up. The risk of either type of tumour following partial mole is much smaller.

The point of surgical evacuation following molar

pregnancy is to remove all the trophoblastic tissue; but it is difficult to be sure that it has all been removed. Thirty years ago one just had to guess and hope. Today, the story is different. After surgery, blood levels of hCG fall to non-pregnant levels quite quickly – for nearly half of cases, within a couple of months. If hCG fails to fall, or even rises during this time, it must mean that some trophoblast remains, either in the womb or perhaps in another site outside the womb, like the pelvis or lungs, to which it has escaped via the bloodstream. Thus it is that weekly, and later monthly and then two-monthly blood checks for hCG, are essential for follow-up. Because pregnancy would mask any sinister rise in hCG levels, women must use effective contraception (usually a low dose oestrogen pill) during the follow-up period, and avoid pregnancy.

All women who have had a molar pregnancy are registered through the Royal College of Obstetricians and Gynaecologists. Three centres in Britain (Charing Cross Hospital, London, Ninewells Hospital, Dundee and Jessop Hospital, Sheffield) run a postal follow-up service whereby, at appropriate intervals, containers for urine are sent to the patient who returns a sample for analysis. The results are sent back to the patients' consultants or GPs. The three units endeavour to ensure that no patient is lost to follow-up.

It is important to stress that 90 per cent of women will have nothing but negative results. For cases where there has been partial mole and hCG levels have fallen to normal 56 days later, follow-up may only be necessary for six months at most, before trying again for a baby. The standard follow-up time, however, is two years, and no case of GTT has been identified after completing a two-year follow-up. For the majority of women, not getting pregnant for two years is probably no hardship. But for some, especially those who are older, this wait may feel like a life sentence. Enough is known, however, for obstetricians to be flexible, providing women know the risks. For instance, women whose hCG levels only fall to normal more than 56 days after evacuation, and whose levels then remain normal for a subsequent six months, still have a risk of 1 in 286 of developing GTT. In these cases if women want to go ahead with pregnancy the choice is theirs; the odds are heavily in their favour. In comparison, a woman aged 36 and 9 months at the time of delivery, has the same risk of having a baby with Down's Syndrome. It might make a 36-year-old woman stop and think, and have appropriate testing, but would it stop her having a baby? I might add that 1 in 200 is the risk of death at the same age if you smoke more than 20 cigarettes a day and you may know a lot of women who run this sort of risk without concern.

Because trophoblast tissue can get into the mother's bloodstream, it can spread, as I have said, to other sites in the body (metastasis), usually the lungs or pelvis. If it is in these sites it is very amenable to treatment with specialist drugs which will be given in different combinations, depending on whether a woman is low, medium or high risk.

Very high hCG levels at the time of evacuation or in the subsequent four weeks will prompt chemotherapy. Low risk therapy is short, will not cause hair loss and has a cure rate of virtually 100 per cent. Medium risk therapy involves a short cycle of treatment (3–4 weeks) and there may be some hair loss. High risk treatment is for those for whom previous treatment has failed.

Coping

If you have a complete mole, and know that there never was a baby, it can be very difficult; you have been pregnant, and yet

you weren't – at least not in the conventional sense. Nevertheless, pregnancy and a baby were what you were expecting
and these expectations have suddenly been removed in a
dramatic, and at first, an incomprehensible way. And now, to
make things worse, you have been told that you may not get
pregnant for some time yet. Molar pregnancy is so hard to
explain that you may be justified in saying to people that you
simply had a miscarriage and don't feel like trying again for a
while. But you have been fortunate to escape a condition
which used to be a killer.

11

Pre-eclampsia

'Why hadn't I heard of pre-eclampsia?'

'I was astonished when I heard how common pre-eclampsia is.'

'I never realised just how dangerous it was, not just to the baby but me too.'

If there were three chapters in this book that I could insist that all pregnant women read, they would be on caesarean section, on premature delivery and on pre-eclampsia. Each affects about one in ten pregnancies, making them very common, yet everyone assumes that prematurity and sections are things that happen to other women – and nobody's ever heard of pre-eclampsia. It wasn't a bit surprising to find that they were the three major complications of pregnancy mentioned in the 'I wish I'd known' section. In this and the subsequent chapters, I describe why they happen and the implications.

Alarming medical details tend, when they are written for the general public, to come hand in hand with information about how such frightening outcomes can be prevented. When you are already pregnant, there is not much you can do about prevention. If you were into prevention, you would have chosen celibacy. You might like to read this and the following chapters in the same way that you might read a first aid manual. When doing so, you fervently hope that you will never see someone having a heart attack, but if you did, you would be very glad that you knew how to cope and what to do. The feelings of bystanders faced with medical emergency such as heart attack are often those of helplessness, of panic, and confusion about what they should do for the best. From our survey, much the same feelings were faced by those who experienced the major complications of childbearing. 'If only I'd known', they all said. Well, here is the information, but be rational about it. Remember the first aid manual – whilst sensibly preparing yourself for the worst, you are able to put things in perspective and realise that the next person you meet will not fall to the ground, requiring your newly acquired first aid skills.

Pre-eclampsia is the commonest, and potentially most serious, complication of pregnancy, affecting 1 in 10 women, yet there's a good chance that you may not even have heard of it. It is characterised by a range of symptoms of which the three best known are high blood pressure, swelling (oedema) and protein in the urine (proteinuria). Over 50,000 pregnancies a year are affected by pre-eclampsia. It is the single largest cause of maternal mortality, killing about 10 women a year in Britain and thousands more worldwide. In the UK, it also causes the death of nearly 1,000 babies annually and many more babies are born smaller than they should be because of it.

Given these gobsmacking statistics, why isn't pre-eclampsia better known? And why do so few pregnancy manuals even mention it? Part of the problem is the reluctance, as we have seen, of professionals to impart bad news about pregnancy. Another part is, despite decades of concentrated research, that the disease is so poorly understood. The other factor is, I believe, its name. Many years ago, it was called toxaemia (a name which may be more familiar to you) because it was thought (erroneously) to be caused by a toxin in the mother's blood. But there are many other names; for instance, pregnancy-induced hypertension (PIH), pre-eclamptic toxaemia (PET), pregnancy-associated hypertension (PAH) or even hypertensive disease of pregnancy (HDP). If the professionals can't agree on what to call it, no wonder women are confused. For the purposes of this chapter, pre-eclampsia is used to describe the condition which is specific to pregnancy, which can lead to a more serious form of the condition which may include the mother having fits (eclampsia) and which is characterised by a group of signs of which high blood pressure (hypertension) is one.

Who Gets It?

Pre-eclampsia is, therefore, more than just having high blood pressure. Before telling you more about it, who does it affect? In the main it affects first pregnancies, and although it is possible to get it in a second pregnancy most women who develop pre-eclampsia in a first pregnancy will not suffer a recurrence, or if they do it may not be as severe. Only very rarely indeed will a woman have a first brush with pre-eclampsia in a second pregnancy, and sometimes this happens because there has been a change of partner, for reasons which will become clearer as you read on. Pre-eclampsia runs in families, so if your mother or sisters suffered from it you are more likely to suffer from it. Being older, being of short stature, having pre-existing medical conditions, particularly chronic hypertension or kidney disease, or having a multiple pregnancy are all risk factors. Molar pregnancy (see Chapter 10) is strongly linked with pre-eclampsia. Pregnancy complications are notorious for their association with social class but this condition affects all social classes equally, rich and poor, nourished and malnourished. It is not affected by smoking.

Causes

The risk list above gives some clues about the causes of pre-eclampsia. It has an inherited component and the search for the relevant gene or genes is currently in full swing. There is another element as well. Pre-eclampsia is not as common in second and subsequent pregnancies. This pattern is rather like that seen with infectious disease – once you've had mumps, for instance, you are unlikely to get it again, or if you do, not to the same degree. This would suggest an immune factor and certainly, as witnessed by the huge numbers of immune system cells in the developing placenta in early pregnancy, the immune system is very heavily involved in the establishment of healthy pregnancy. Further weight is added to this by the knowledge that a change of partner can precipitate pre-eclampsia in a new pregnancy, sometimes despite several previous unaffected pregnancies, rather in the same way that the 'newness' of a recently mutated cold virus can cause a cold, even though you have only just had one.

The disease is only cured once the baby is delivered, which suggests that the baby is the cause. However, molar pregnancy, in which there is no baby, just a collection of cells of placental origin, is strongly linked to pre-eclampsia, suggesting that it is not the baby but the placenta which is the culprit.

The best known diagnostic symptoms of pre-eclampsia appear in the second half of pregnancy, but the foundations for the disease are laid very soon after conception, probably before you are even aware that you are having a baby.

The fertilised egg is surrounded by a double envelope of

cells. These specialised cells are called trophoblast and they have a vital role, firstly in nourishing the early embryo and then in the formation of the placenta. When the fertilised egg sinks into the lining of the womb, the trophoblast cells in contact with the womb lining start to burrow into it. And here is the first dilemma. The cells of your baby are different to yours – in fact if you had a kidney transplant of your baby's tissue type, you'd reject it in a couple of weeks. The body's defence system, the immune system, is programmed to seek and destroy anything which it recognises as not being 'self'. This should mean death and destruction for those burrowing trophoblast cells – yet somehow, not only they but the developing baby (which you would have thought was an absolute giveaway in the foreign body stakes) escape its attention.

The trophoblast cells have two jobs now. One is to form the placenta, the other is to do some structural engineering work on the blood vessels in the womb lining so that they can carry sufficient blood to keep the growing baby supplied, via the placenta, with oxygen and nutrients. Trophoblast cells invade the coiled blood vessels (the spiral arterioles) of the womb lining, breaking down their walls and transforming them from tight tubes to big, floppy, funnel-shaped vessels, capable of taking not just 50 ml of blood per minute (the normal flow), but 800 ml of blood per minute. In women who have pre-eclampsia this process of infiltration by trophoblast cells seems to be limited in some way – perhaps because the immune system has recognised and stopped some, if not all, of the cells from doing their job properly. In fact the infiltration process, which eventually makes these blood vessels capable of carrying 100 times their normal volume of blood, and which normally goes on until about 18 weeks, seems to stop at about 12 weeks in women who have pre-eclampsia.

The consequences of this 'sick' placenta are far reaching. The presence of the placenta tells the body that it needs to adapt its systems in preparation for pregnancy. These adaptations are spectacular in their scope: for instance, there is a nearly 50 per cent increase in blood volume, body water increases by up to 8.5 litres and the blood clots more easily (this latter is to ensure that you do not bleed to death when the placenta is delivered). The signals that come from a 'sick' placenta, particularly as the pregnancy progresses, cause some of the body's systems to react, rather than adapt, in a way that is potentially life-threatening to both mother and developing baby. For instance, signals that cause blood vessels to constrict result in an increased blood pressure, but also mean a decrease in bloodflow through the placenta which is the baby's lifeline. I should point out here that whilst the mother's blood pressure can affect the baby's wellbeing, it does not cause damage to the baby, nor does the baby itself develop high blood pressure.

Blood Pressure

Although blood pressure is a very familiar term, its mechanics are, I guess, pretty much a haze for most of us. Understanding blood pressure, however, is the key to understanding pre-eclampsia; so, wrap the wet towel around the head and concentrate on the next couple of paragraphs.

As I have said, there is a dramatic increase in blood volume in pregnancy. Because of all this extra blood, the heart has to work harder and cardiac output (the amount of blood pumped out with each heartbeat) increases by 30 per cent. Each beat of the heart forces blood through the arteries. On page 63 I explained how readings are given as two figures, one above the other, and how doctors are more concerned by the bottom one, the diastolic reading recorded when the heart relaxes between beats.

Blood pressure is determined partly by the cardiac output and partly by the state of the blood and arteries. If the blood is thick, and the arteries are small and narrow, more pressure is required in order to force the blood through the vessels. If you find this mystifying, think about it like this. You are given a garden hose and are asked to clean two muddy drainpipes, one narrow, one wide. Just putting the hose in the wide one is sufficient to wash the mud out, but to clean the narrow pipe as effectively you would probably need to squeeze the end of the hose – thereby increasing the pressure of the water – in order to force the mud and water through the narrow bore of the pipe. If cardiac output increases and the blood is thicker in pregnancy, blood pressure ought to rise. In fact, blood pressure either remains the same or falls, particularly in the early months. This is because the blood vessels are far more relaxed and floppy, making it easier for blood to flow through them (the technical term is less resistant).

The placenta produces a substance called prostacyclin which helps achieve this. However, it also produces thromboxane, a hormone-like compound which has directly the opposite effect: it can constrict blood vessels and activate platelets – the specialised blood cells involved in the clotting process. In women with pre-eclampsia, the placenta produces three times as much thromboxane as a normal placenta, and only half as much prostacyclin – so, unlike in normal pregnancies, the effect of thromboxane predominates. With thicker blood, and with arteries being constricted, blood pressure must rise in women with pre-eclampsia if blood is to continue to flow properly.

The thromboxane story isn't, however, the whole picture. If it were, one might have expected a considerable reduction in the incidence of pre-eclampsia with low-dose aspirin (aspirin suppresses thromboxane production), but the results of the CLASP trial (of which more later) showed that for most women there was not. In some ways thinking about how the secondary symptoms of pre-eclampsia are caused have come full circle. You will remember that pre-eclampsia used to be called toxaemia because it was thought that the disease resulted from the presence of a toxin in the blood. Recent research has concentrated on a similar theory – that there is an X factor, produced by the placenta, which when released into the circulation causes the familiar secondary symptoms of the disease. Very recently indeed a substance has been identified which might well be that elusive factor X. This substance is of interest because it has such a dramatic effect on the specialised cells – called endothelial cells – which line blood vessels. In fact, it is so potent that even a small amount literally strips the endothelial cells away, causing the blood vessels to become damaged and leaky. Leaking blood vessels would also account for the other two classic symptoms seen in pre-eclamptic women – oedema and proteinuria.

When blood vessels become leaky, water seeps out of them and fills every available nook and cranny round about. Water retained in this way is difficult for the body to excrete. Since water is so heavy, women who retain it will inevitably put on a lot of weight. The fluid retention is often most noticeable in the ankles and fingers, but the whole body is affected. Normally if you press your thumb on, say, your arm, no dent remains when you remove your thumb. If fluid is being retained, a dent will remain until the water that has been displaced by the pressure of your thumb returns – usually several seconds later; and this can be seen at almost any site on the body. Fluid retention is very common, even in perfectly healthy pregnancies, and by itself it is not a symptom of pre-eclampsia (nor is it, incidentally, invariably associated with it).

Another consequence of 'leaky' blood vessels is damage to the body's filtering mechanisms in the kidneys. Instead of retaining useful proteins in the blood, the kidneys allow small amounts of protein to escape into the urine. Proteinuria, particularly if allied to blood pressure and oedema, should never ever be regarded as a trivial symptom, for it is a sign that pre-eclampsia is developing to an unstable advanced stage. When protein consistently appears in the urine, the pregnancy has a strictly limited life – for some women it may be as much as six weeks, for others it may be as little as two days. The average is fourteen days, and if delivery is not achieved before this time, pre-eclampsia runs a good chance of moving into its third and most advanced stage, eclampsia.

Treatment

So how is this to be prevented? Nothing can be done to prevent the first stage of pre-eclampsia, which occurs at the very beginning of a pregnancy. But good antenatal care should spot the symptoms of the second stage, particularly those of raised blood pressure and proteinuria which can both be measured in an objective way. Providing these signs are spotted and action taken to deliver the baby early, thus pre-empting serious illness, the vast majority of mothers have nothing further to fear, either for themselves or their babies. Thus it is that the whole of antenatal care is geared towards the detection of this one disease, with urine, blood pressure and weight being carefully recorded at each visit. Yet how many women know the importance of these measurements – or what they are for?

If you have raised blood pressure and proteinuria, or any

other symptoms of pre-eclampsia, and hospital admission is suggested, you may feel fairly desperate about it, particularly if you have other children to care for. You may say things like, 'Couldn't I rest at home?' in an effort to avoid being taken in. Again there is a myth here, which is that you are being admitted to hospital for bed rest, and that bed rest is somehow a cure for pre-eclampsia. It isn't. The point about taking you in to hospital is that pre-eclampsia is a very unpredictable disease; you are there in order that your vital signs, and those of the baby, can be closely monitored, because nobody is able to tell at this stage what is going to happen next. The only sure thing is that pre-eclampsia is a progressive condition, and once you have proteinuria the countdown clock has started ticking – except nobody knows how much time there is left on the clock. That's why you need to be in hospital.

> 'They say I nearly died. All I remember was how well I felt.'

> 'I couldn't understand what all the fuss was about, I felt blooming.'

All of this may seem very hard, particularly if, like most other women with pre-eclampsia, you are feeling perfectly well – blooming, indeed – which makes it all the more difficult for you to appreciate that there is something seriously wrong. You may fight hospital admission, and this is natural when you feel on top of the world. Very few people actively want to go into hospital, but you have a disease which is potentially life-threatening and you cannot be held in any sort of safety net anywhere other than a fully equipped hospital, which can take those pre-emptive measures which might be necessary to save your baby and possibly even you, such as an emergency delivery by section. Don't fight it.

If there is one thing the medical profession likes to do, it is to put diseases in pigeonholes. Pre-eclampsia refuses to be boxed up in this way. The onset of symptoms can start as early as 20 weeks, or not appear until 40 weeks, or appear anywhere in between. There is no single definitive test that will tell doctors that a woman has pre-eclampsia, only a bewildering range of symptoms from which to make deductions. Although raised blood pressure is the best known symptom, women can have severe pre-eclampsia without their blood pressure being raised. On the other hand, their blood pressure may be astronomic but their pre-eclampsia very mild. There is no specific treatment for the condition, and certainly no cure, unless you count delivery of the baby as a cure. And women themselves aren't even aware of the condition, because they feel perfectly well. Is it any wonder that pre-eclampsia is so little known? Or that, in retrospect, so many of the same mistakes are made time and time again in diagnosing, or rather not diagnosing the disease.

Talking to obstetricians, you quickly become aware that severe cases of eclampsia, whilst all too familiar to an older generation of doctors, are simply not seen by younger ones, mainly because of the improvements in antenatal care, which have made a difficult condition not just confusing in its presentation but unfamiliar too. The main mistake for doctors is not to take a rise in blood pressure seriously and to treat it as being due to nervousness, overwork, exhaustion etc, etc. And, having told you that the bottom figure of a blood pressure measurement (the diastolic reading) is the more important one – which in general it is – doctors tend to believe their own press and fall into the trap of discounting a very high systolic (such as 170), just because the bottom figure is below that magic cut off number of 90. The presence of protein is sometimes dismissed if it is associated with mild hypertension, and the condition labelled as mild pre-eclampsia, when in fact all pre-eclampsia is severe and should be treated as an emergency for same-day admission. The sudden onset of jaundice or upper abdominal pain (which may arise because of liver complications) or severe vomiting in pregnancy should not be dismissed as trivial (although the latter are very common symptoms) without proper investigation as all can be symptoms of pre-eclampsia. I say all this because time and time again, eclampsia has not been pre-empted as it should and has been allowed to get out of hand simply because those warning signs were not recognised. This was often the case even when a woman was clearly giving her carers an ominous list of symptoms which somebody should have spotted immediately as having pre-eclampsia written all over them.

In many pregnancy books, the symptoms of impending eclampsia are given as headache, flashing lights, visual disturbances, etc. It shouldn't ever get to this stage – believe me, your body has been shouting the odds long before. So, listen to your body and if it's shouting, make sure you shout too. And if you have a blood pressure of 140/90 with the new appearance of proteinuria (plus one or more) expect to be admitted to hospital the same day, don't fight it and if you are not admitted, ask why not. I am conscious of having been horribly bossy here – I know that the last thing most women want to do is cause a fuss – especially when they may feel perfectly well, but I also know that there will be women who will thank me for this advice in years to come.

Close monitoring will be the order of the day if you are admitted to hospital. Although delivery may be the only cure, it may not be appropriate if you are less than 36 weeks gestation. If blood pressure rises suddenly to 170 mmHg systolic or 110 mmHg diastolic, expect to be given medication to reduce your blood pressure. If blood pressure is allowed to rise unchecked, it has the potential to cause dangerously unpredictable medical emergencies, such as cerebral haemorrhage caused by arteries bursting. You should be aware, however, that stroke-inducing blood pressures are in the order of 200/130 mmHg – so there is a very wide margin of safety. Nevertheless, the aim is to get it under some sort of control, especially if the rise has been very sudden, when fast acting anti-hypertensive drugs such as hydralzine may be given. However the disadvantage of this drug is that it mimics some of the symptoms of impending eclampsia, such as severe headache and can only be administered by injection. Another type of acute control drug is a calcium channel blocker called nifedipine (the most familiar brand name is Adalat) which can be given orally but also causes headache. These drugs are for acute symptoms but if you are at a relatively early stage of pregnancy, then other drugs must be given which can lower the blood pressure systematically over a longer period of time – the point being to give the baby a bit more time in the womb. There are a range of drugs of which methyldopa and beta-blockers are the most common. Methyldopa (brand names Aldomet, Dopamet, etc) is known to be a safe drug for use in pregnancy, although it initially causes sedation, and then tiredness. Beta-blockers, such as labetalol, cause fewer side effects and although they have not been used as widely as methyldopa, their short term safety for the baby is well documented.

You may be given medicine to prevent convulsions, such as diazepam (Valium). Some hospitals prescribe this to all women they deem at risk but others are more selective, preferring to give drugs such as phenytoin (a drug more usually given to epileptics) or magnesium sulphate which is widely used in the States on an individual basis. Once fitting has occurred, even if it is controlled, the risk of more fits is great and urgent delivery is essential. The severest form of eclampsia is terrifying for doctors, carers and especially a woman's partner – individual body systems such as the kidneys or liver may fail and the woman may be moved into the hospital's intensive care unit. Luckily the woman herself is unlikely to be aware of what is going on.

You might think that, once the baby has been delivered, the immediate danger is past but it is possible to have convulsions as much as six days after delivery and for this reason expect to be very closely supervised and cosseted. After the birth, blood pressure rises steadily during the first five days and this trend can be exaggerated if you have had pre-eclampsia, so you may be given beta-blockers. Your blood pressure should be closely monitored for at least three weeks after delivery and, although you may have been allowed to go home long before this time, you may well continue to receive medication for a minimum of a couple of weeks.

Even though you may have sustained damage to some of your organs, such as liver or kidney at the height of the crisis, this is normally reversible and, for the vast majority of women, there will be no long-term effects. It may be, however, that further investigation will reveal a kidney problem or under-lying hypertension which aggravated the disease and which was not known at the start of your pregnancy. Having had pre-eclampsia does not necessarily mean that you will have blood pressure problems yourself in later life, although this is evidently not the case if you already had high blood pressure before pregnancy. Many women who have had pre-eclampsia therefore will have hypertension in later life.

Your baby may be smaller than normal – in effect, she has

been starved of the necessary nutrients because of poor blood flow through the placenta. Being little may mean that she needs additional care at birth, even if you reach a stage of pregnancy at which other women are having hulks. Growth-retarded babies tend to put on weight quickly, however, once born, and soon catch up. If your baby has also been delivered early, she may have additional problems of prematurity (see chapter 15).

Coping

Of all pregnancy complications, I personally think this one is one of the most difficult to cope with. For a start, despite how common it is, nobody has heard of pre-eclampsia. Nobody appreciates how sick you are, because you may look and feel perfectly well, and therefore nobody, least of all you, is prepared for the lightning descent into crisis that it can precipitate. Because it can constitute a full-blown medical emergency, doctors may sometimes be reluctant to talk about the consequences of the disease for fear of frightening you. In some ways this can be completely counterproductive because you will pick up the staff's (unvoiced) concerns and end up being even more alarmed. Other doctors can be brutally honest – as I fear I may have been above – to the point of being insensitive. The middle path is one in which doctors communicate with you and discuss their concerns and how they propose to manage the problem with you and your partner, involving you fully in your care. However, you have to accept that, sometimes, the very speed of onset will necessarily make you an onlooker rather than a participant in your care.

I think the overwhelming feeling I have from talking to

women who have had severe pre-eclampsia is one of lack of
control. Frequently what they say is peppered with little
comments like 'and I never smoked' or 'I was really fit', as if
somehow the fact that they had been sensible and prepared for
pregnancy ought to have protected them in some way. What
no one ever tells women is that the vast majority of pregnancy
problems can neither be predicted nor be prevented by diet,
by good health or being fit – which is why women should not
believe that they are the guilty party when pregnancy goes
wrong. Women who have had pre-eclampsia are sometimes
the most guilty mothers of all, believing that they must have
been at fault in some way – nothing could be further from the
truth.

Don't expect to get over a crisis pregnancy quickly. It may
take you months or even years. You may feel cheated because
your delivery was nothing like the one that you had planned
and you will certainly, as I have said, feel guilty and bewildered
by your experience. In addition to having to cope with an
extremely serious illness yourself, you may have a baby in
special care and the prospect of months of uncertainty and
anxiety with the scale of intensive treatment required. You
may have experienced the worst of all worlds – having had
many months in hospital or a sudden dramatically shocking
end to your pregnancy, only to lose your baby at the end. You
may find yourself facing a conflicting range of emotions – grief
at the loss of your baby but, knowing how ill you were, relief
at the same time. These opposing feelings may make you feel
very wretched and you may not want to talk to, or see, other
mothers for a while.

It is important, I think, that you try and share your
experiences with someone – either someone who is a trained
counsellor or perhaps with another mother who has been
through the same thing (try contacting one through APEC,

see the Appendix). Above all, you should talk to your doctor, again and again if necessary, so that you really understand what happened. I should also mention that it is common to blame medical staff, particularly if early signs were not spotted, for the way in which your pregnancy ended. They should have been more alert, but you should be aware that that may not have made a difference to the outcome of pregnancy in your case.

You will probably also have a partner who is completely shell-shocked by the whole experience. You were at least out of it — he was the one who was told that your life was on the line. He will need almost as much support as you but may not be able to articulate his need for help. On a lighter note — because this is getting very serious — sometimes in melodramas you get the 'Who shall I save? Mother or baby?' question asked by doctors of the prospective father. Although the condition is never mentioned by name, pre-eclampsia is the problem and it is true that in extreme cases delivery has to take place in the sure and certain knowledge that the baby will not survive at such an early gestation.

Trying again

As I have indicated, pre-eclampsia is a disease that can be pre-empted but not prevented in the true sense of the word. However, a number of people still make claims to the contrary. First off, diet. Because salt restriction is advised for people with blood pressure problems, it is assumed that it will be helpful for women with pre-eclampsia. In the only large trial of this, women on salt-restricted diets fared worse than women on normal diets. In the Eighties, a doctor called Thomas Brewer claimed that pre-eclampsia is a disease of malnutrition (partly because pre-eclampsia is accompanied by low levels of protein in the blood) and that it is entirely preventable with a proper balanced diet. Giving pregnant women high protein supplements does not reduce the incidence of pre-eclampsia, and in fact causes a reduction in the baby's birthweight which is potentially very harmful, even more so if the baby is also smaller than it should be because of the mother's pre-eclampsia. The fact that the condition strikes rich and poor with equal ferocity should tell you immediately that diet is not central to pre-eclampsia, although it may modify other factors responsible for the condition.

An attempt by the People's League of Health in 1942 to supplement pregnant women's diets showed a decrease in pre-eclampsia. At the time it wasn't clear which element of the supplement was responsible for the fall in pre-eclampsia. The spotlight fell on cod liver oil because firstly Faroese Islanders (who have a diet rich in fish) have a low incidence of the disease, and because fatty acids, which are present in large quantity in fish oils, are involved in the clotting process and might reasonably have a role in ameliorating some of the effects of pre-eclampsia. Although this has yet to be substantiated, there are two caveats. Studies of families in Iceland and Scotland have identified families in which there is a very strong history of the disease and it could simply be that the Faroe Islands have a low incidence of the gene, or genes involved in the disease, within their population. The second is that fish oils contain high quantities of Vitamin A which is known to cause birth defects, so you should approach supplementation with fish oils with great caution. The other element to excite current interest is calcium. Studies in Ecuador, in areas with low calcium intake, have shown a remarkable decrease in disease incidence with calcium supplementation.

Women who have pre-eclampsia tend to put on a great

deal of weight during pregnancy, so it was assumed that they were overeating and that excessive weight gain was the cause of the pre-eclampsia. As explained elsewhere, it is now known that weight gain is a consequence of pre-eclampsia – water is retained and quite simply, water weighs a lot – not its cause. Drugs that force the body to expel water – diuretics – were used in the past as it was believed that retained fluid was an early sign of pre-eclampsia and that treatment with diuretics would help in prevention. It doesn't.

Women who have existing hypertension are known to be at particular risk of pre-eclampsia and it would seem logical that controlling their blood pressure in early pregnancy with drugs might reduce the incidence of the disease. This has not proved to be the case.

A while ago, there were a number of reports in the scientific literature regarding low dose aspirin (a quarter to a fifth of a normal tablet) which really seemed to help prevent the disease. Very good results indeed were achieved in some trials and there was great excitement that here, at last, was the preventive treatment that everyone had been looking for. However, hopes were dashed with the publication of the multinational CLASP trial. Tens of thousands of women were involved but the results showed that there was hardly any difference at all in outcome in those women who had received low dose aspirin compared to those who had received placebo. It was a bitterly disappointing result and one that could not be ignored.

I think that the most helpful thing I can say to you is to make sure that before your next pregnancy, you get your GP to refer you to an expert in pre-eclampsia – probably at a teaching hospital. Talking to someone who is an expert in the condition may relieve many of your worries. They may be prepared to take you on. Alternatively, they may advise your local hospital. Certainly a key element in prevention is making sure that you are scrupulously monitored in your next pregnancy.

So if pre-eclampsia is not preventable, what will happen next time around? My good friend Chris Redman, one of the world's leading authorities on pre-eclampsia and about as sensible and humane a doctor as you are ever likely to meet, sums up the situation thus: 'The chances of pre-eclampsia occurring again are not as great as some mothers would think but more than they would like.' It is not right that if you have had pre-eclampsia in a first pregnancy that you will definitely not get it again. However, the good news is that the chance of a severe recurrence is about 1 in 20 and if you don't get it in a subsequent pregnancy, the risk thereafter is very low indeed. Your risk if you have other predisposing conditions such as chronic high blood pressure, a change of partner, kidney disease or multiple pregnancy needs to be expertly assessed. It is not true either that if you have never had pre-eclampsia, that you cannot get it in a subsequent pregnancy – this happens unaccountably to about 1 in 150 women.

In the future it may be possible to predict the disease with greater certainty and since 9 out of 10 women do not suffer from it, it would mean a reduction in the level of antenatal care required for most women – and a welcome increase in surveillance for those known to be at risk. It might be possible to detect women who were genetically most at risk – although it is likely that several genes, including some in the baby, are at work, rather than just one, which would make things tricky as far as testing was concerned. There is some evidence that alterations in platelet activity in early pregnancy might provide a good early test and there is progress towards identification of the mysterious factor released by the placenta which causes such a devastating effect on so many body systems.

Pre-eclampsia is one of the most contradictory diseases known to man. As I said, it refuses to be pigeonholed and has defeated scientists who attempt to find either its cause or more importantly a cure. I predict that it will remain a disease of contradiction for many years to come but that knowledge of its effects is, for the present, the surest route to good health for mother and baby.

12

Labour

I had a hunch before I started this book that women were very often not prepared for what actually happened during their labours, and this was borne out by our survey. We asked women who had already had children whether, with hindsight, they were prepared for what actually happened during their deliveries. An astonishing 42 per cent said that they were not. Even amongst those women who had had two children or more, the proportion who felt adequately prepared was only 51 per cent. What's going wrong?

Perhaps the most important point to make is that not only do labours differ between one woman and another, but they can be radically different from one delivery to another in the same woman. Most labours have three recognisable stages, during the second of which a baby or babies are delivered. Most books present this admirable plan without adding the essential bit of information – that there is infinite scope for variety and drama within this basic plot and there ain't no advance warning of your own storyline. Thus you are prepared for a 'standard' labour, but in truth there is no such thing – much in the same way as there is no such thing as a standard size 12, or condoms that come in small sizes. Some women in our survey hinted as much when they said that the reason for them being unprepared was that 'nothing can prepare you for the unknown'.

But the unknown is an awfully scary concept. In some

ways, women have come to an awkward halfway house in the knowledge stakes. It is better for them to know than not know, but don't whatever you do tell them too much because you'll scare them half to death is the general gist of it. Thus it is that women are taught the sanitised Laura Ashley version of labour – and very often come unstuck because, for instance, they are not prepared for a premature birth, caesarean section or an induced birth – three of the commonest variations of 'standard' (all of which are discussed in separate chapters). You might already be feeling alarmed in case these things happen to you. You might be one of those women who have left pregnancy fairly late and have thus heard every labour horror story under the sun. You might just be worried about how you'll cope with an ordinary labour, let alone anything out of the ordinary and have been feeling a rising sense of panic. And yet here I am trying to hold your hand and prepare you – no wonder so many books have stuck to the rosy glow version of labour. But if I did that, I'd be failing you. The first thing to say, and very firmly, is that just because you read about it, doesn't mean that you will experience it. The problem is – and it applies as much to the minor indignities and difficulties that women told us about, such as cramp and nausea and the shakes – that if you do experience these things, and you haven't heard about them, you'll think you are the only one this is happening to, a complete freak and failure, not to mention frightened. And being frightened is in itself a way of racking up the pain and panic points.

'I felt out of control.' I lost count of the number of women that wept on my shoulder during my years at WellBeing on the general subject of labour – 'It all went wrong, I felt out of control.' The usual problem was that women had decided in advance what sort of labour they would have, either on the basis of previous labours or from some idealised view of the birth process. These are always dangerous waters because, as I have indicated, the exact course of labour cannot be predicted. And it follows that if something is unpredictable, you cannot control it in the conventional sense of the word. Expecting to be able to control labour is a bit like expecting to be in control of a runaway horse – all right in a nice quiet field but hopeless if you've got a fire engine racing past you at the same time. You can't be in control of a haemorrhage, neither can you control fetal distress, and you can't control the length of your labour much either. The 'I felt out of control' most commonly came from women who had decided that they would have natural deliveries without pain relief who then, through no fault of their own, had long, difficult labours or some other labour drama. They became exhausted and many ended up having forceps or other interventions, not to mention pain relief (usually everything going and more besides). They were bitterly disappointed that their labour wasn't as they had expected.

I was always struck when I spoke to these women by their overpowering sense of failure, as if by not having a 'natural' birth they were somehow a lesser woman or a bad mother. Having a baby will probably be the single most memorable experience in your life. For me, it ranked up there with falling in love for the first time and my wedding day as being heart-burstingly, dizzyingly happy. It's having the baby that makes you happy but the whole experience that affects you. The baby is lifelong happiness; the experience of labour is strictly time limited. Birth is a balance between your quality of experience and the need to ensure that your baby is born healthy. The two are not, and never have been, mutually incompatible. It should be perfectly possible, and the aim of all your medical carers, to combine them, but you need to be open-minded and flexible and accept that there is an infinite variety of 'good births' to be had, in which the key element is not whether you did or did not have pain relief, or did or did not have a 'normal' delivery, but whether you felt positive and secure and were safely delivered of a healthy baby. For that you need to know all the options, and to have no fixed ideas in advance of how it's going to be. Trust me.

For the purposes of this chapter, I am assuming that the majority of you will give birth in a hospital or GP unit setting.

Preparing for Labour

'I was so enthusiastic about packing a bag first time round – I never used half the stuff I took – it was all quite different the second time.'

People differ enormously in what they feel they need to take with them to hospital. If you read Chapter 17, 'After the Birth', you'll get a good feel for what you might need for your stay. You might also have some ideas about what you will need during labour and I would advise packing these separately, not only so that you don't have to rummage through your case to find them all, but also so that they can be taken home by your partner separately when labour is over.

You may have decided on the hospital option but still want to make it as personalised and home-like an experience as you can – so wearing your own clothes, or even nothing, during labour may be important to you. On the other hand, you're likely to end up wrecking your own nightie or shirt, and although a hospital gown isn't glamourous it's certainly practical and someone else does the laundry. Take nighties that button down the front so you don't have to pull your clothes over your head when you're examined or when you're breast feeding. Men's shirts are brilliant. And take lots of them – you'll get through more nighties than you thought was possible; at least one a day. Take disposable knickers and a supply of maternity sanitary towels (very few hospitals provide more than a token few these days).

It will help you feel less like a patient if you dress normally during the day. So take some ordinary clothes that are fairly loose fitting, and whatever you do don't pack depression in denim – by which I mean, don't pack the jeans you wore before you got pregnant. Your tummy doesn't disappear that quickly; in fact, you'll carry on looking fairly pregnant for several days. There's no way you'll get your jeans on, and if you can, just keep quiet, because we hate you already. You will need your maternity bras, together with slippers (floors are usually filthy) and a dressing gown. Finally, remember that maternity hospitals are heated to tropical levels, so don't pack winter-weight stuff, even if it is the middle of winter. That also means, of course, that your partner should come in light clothes when he accompanies you to the delivery room.

For reasons I outline in the 'After the Birth' chapter, take some cleaning stuff – Dettox or the like, plus some cleaning cloths. You will be very thirsty so you might like to take squash or fruit juice (although beware, large quantities of orange juice can upset your baby if you are breast feeding). The peculiarities of hospital catering may mean that you have to endure long periods without food when you are starving – e.g. you've had your baby after the evening meal has been served, meaning no food until breakfast time – so you may like to pack some sort of snack food. Little boxes of cereal are good comfort food snacks – but beware of packing too many biscuits and sweets.

Many hospitals have places where you can make a cup of tea or a slice of toast. Some hospitals will allow you to bring in food. There was an Indian lady in my ward whose husband brought in the most wonderful selection of goodies every night. I thought about asking him to marry me there and then as I contemplated the 'swish it about and it disappears' pink mousse and the minute but solid piece of fish that hospital catering (who are intent on feeding the sick, not the ravenously healthy) had delivered to my bed. Another point regarding food is that the hospital canteen may not be open during the hours that you are in labour, and although you might not want anything your partner or birth companion will, so pack something separately in the snack department for them. I am conscious of having gone on about food rather a lot, but being hungry or thirsty at a time like this is pretty miserable.

Another category of things to pack is related to telling everyone about the baby – pens, birth announcement cards, a list of phone numbers of people to call, as well as phone cards or change for the phones. (You should note that many hospitals do not allow the use of mobile phones because they can affect medical equipment.) In general, don't take anything valuable like purse and credit cards into hospital with you. Pack something diverting to read or do – preferably something light. This is not the moment to try reading Proust. Finally, think of yourself – a sponge bag with your favourite soap or shower gel, shampoo and make-up can be wondrous pick-me-ups, as can things that remind you of home, like a photo of your other child or children.

The most exciting thing of course is bits for the baby. The hospital will usually tell you what is necessary, depending on what they supply in the way of nappies, sleep gowns, etc., but I would suggest that you take a few nappies, a couple of vests or vest bodies, a couple of first size stretch suits, a cardigan, plus, if it is winter, a shawl or wrap and a hat for going home.

Incidentally, I say a couple of vests only because sod's law will dictate that your baby manages to soil whatever you put on her in the first thirty seconds, leaving you nothing but a shawl to wrap her in for her very first journey. You will soon become very experienced about 'spares'. If your partner collects you by car, the car should be equipped with a proper baby seat.

Going into Labour

'I insisted, with this huge great bump, on pulling down a chimney breast. Nesting? It was more like a demolition derby.'

'I had to wash the stairs. Heaven knows why.'

'The last two weeks were bliss, I drifted about, slept and indulged myself.'

'I did more cleaning in two days than I'd ever done in my whole married life.'

'My head was clear and I suddenly had enough energy to go on for hours. My husband said he found me completely exhausting.'

'The baby seemed to drop about two weeks before and then I didn't find breathing such an effort and I was a lot more comfortable, although I seemed to spend every five minutes rushing to the loo.'

Signs of impending labour are many and varied, with the psychological ones being often more noticeable than the physical ones. The pelvis is rather like an old-fashioned tin bucket with a hole in the bottom. The top of the bucket is the pelvic inlet (the widest part of the pelvis), the middle bit is the pelvic cavity and the bottom is the pelvic outlet (the narrowest bit). When the baby is said to be 'engaged', the presenting part (the biggest bit, usually the head) has moved into the bucket (the pelvic outlet). Just how far it has moved into the bucket may be shown on your notes by $\frac{1}{5}$, $\frac{3}{5}$ and finally $\frac{5}{5}$, meaning that your baby's head is one fifth into the bucket and so on, until the head is completely contained within the pelvis. This process begins to happen at about 36 weeks (or even earlier) in first pregnancies and rather later (sometimes not until labour begins) in second and subsequent pregnancies. This accounts for the 'lightening' or dropping which makes you so much more comfortable in the last weeks, particularly if the baby's feet and knees have been kicking the hell out of your ribs. The baby will have more restricted movements as a result and you will almost certainly notice that you empty your bladder more as the baby's head presses down harder and harder on it. This is when mild incontinence is often most likely. You may also be increasingly aware of the baby bouncing on your cervix at this time and walk around feeling as if the baby will literally drop out any second. I was running a Christmas fair the day before my second baby was born and was convinced that he would drop out as I was tacking up tinsel on some stairs, in sight of about 400 people.

As labour draws nearer you may notice a slight loss in weight of up to 3 lbs caused by water loss as hormone levels alter. You might get a bit of diarrhoea or be sick, and put it down to something you ate, when in reality your body is clearing its systems ready for labour. But the most dramatic impending signs may be a sudden burst of manic energy and the 'nesting' instinct. Doctors often poo-poo this; until, that is, they experience it at first hand. It is very difficult to describe. Many women become obsessed with completing a particular task before their baby is born, even when that task is physically very demanding. I insisted on cleaning the windows in our second-floor flat, wedging myself perilously with my bulge hanging right out as I instructed by husband to undertake some other equally ridiculous cleaning ritual. I have a tendency to be bossy, but let me tell you that Margaret Thatcher had nothing on me in those last few days before labour. Men find it very bewildering, torn between indulging you and insisting that you rest. They have a point. You think that you can paper the bedroom, replant your garden, clear out the cupboards, take over the world and then rest prior to labour, but life isn't like this and labour has a knack of catching you out before you get to that all important rest bit. As you will read in chapter 17, overwhelming tiredness is the thing that dominates the first few weeks after the baby's birth and you will end up, as we all do, wishing that you had listened to those nagging voices of experience and rested as you were told. But you may have a sort of St Vitus' dance energy at this stage, together with a feeling of anticipation and excitement that makes rest almost impossible.

For some women, nesting takes the form of endlessly checking their hospital bag, or sorting out the baby's things. You may feel very weary and just want to get the whole thing over with, particularly if you are very uncomfortable. You may feel incredibly relaxed and 'I'm ready for it now', and in the sort of mood where nothing can phase you, nothing worries you and you feel very serene (if you feel like this, treasure the moment, because you'll probably not experience it again for twenty years). But one thing is for sure; you will feel different.

WATERS BREAKING

'As my waters broke, all I could think about was whether I'd have time to shave my legs.'

Hollywood films have a lot to answer for. Contrary to their depiction – one contraction and the baby is there – there is far more time than you think, and the vast majority of women not only have time to shave their legs, but also to shower, wash their hair, have something to eat (see later) and change their clothes, although your partner may take some convincing that this is the case. Most women have at least 10–12 hour first labours. For some reason, many of you wanted to finish the decorating you'd started as well, but I think this is stretching things. If you are going to hospital at night it's probably better to change into day clothes, so that if things come to a halt you can at least feel normal by having ordinary clothes to wear, instead of sauntering about in your teddy bear nightie.

'I wish I'd known that when your waters break, they carry on and on. I thought that they would just gush and stop.'

'It's just as well we'd had new lino put on the bathroom floor, otherwise I would have flooded the flat below when my waters went.'

'I stopped going out in the last couple of weeks because I was so worried that my waters would break in the middle of Boots or something.'

'I wish I'd listened when someone said to put a rubber sheet on the bed. We wrecked ours and it took forever

*to dry out. My husband had to sleep in the spare room
whilst I was in hospital.'*

'Gosh, what a lot.'

For 1 in 10 women, the onset of labour will be heralded by
their waters breaking. Thus it is the exception rather than the
norm. Most women will find that their waters break
spontaneously once labour is well established. There is a lot of
amniotic fluid – up to a litre – so if it all goes at once, it can be
quite dramatic. Amniotic fluid is surprisingly warm, hot even,
with a very characteristic smell. However, it can trickle rather
than gush, depending on exactly where the amniotic sac has
ruptured, and it may be quite tricky to tell whether the wetness
is urine or vaginal secretions instead. Hospitals have test papers
that will show what's what, but a home test is to wipe a bit of
the fluid on a piece of glass and allow it to dry – amniotic fluid
leaves a beautiful ferny pattern, although cervical mucus can
confuse this. Urine will just leave a few crystals.

Normally labour will start spontaneously within a few
hours, but remember that once the waters have broken there is
no barrier against infection for the baby, so be scrupulous
about hygiene when using the loo, have showers rather than
baths, etc. A number of books say solemnly that you shouldn't
make love once the waters have broken. In my view this
statement comes into the same category as the 'have you
thought about contraception?' lady who appears at the bottom
of your bed immediately after delivery: you can't be serious. A
number of women were concerned about possible embarrass-
ment, equating their waters breaking with the ignominy of
publicly wetting yourself. I think you just have to be bold
about this; after all, your bulge will say it all, and as I have
indicated it is much more unlikely than likely to happen.

Besides, people are not very observant and you may well find that no one notices. The point about having a mattress cover is worth making, but most rubber sheets are terribly sweaty to lie on and, given the odds of this happening to you, you may prefer to take the risk.

You don't need to ring the hospital at this stage, providing it is at or within a week or three of term and labour pains follow fairly shortly, although you might like to ring your midwife if this is appropriate to your situation. You do, however, need to tell someone if your waters are not clear but are tinged brown or green (indicating that the baby has passed meconium, its bowel contents, and may be in need of help), or if you know for a fact that the baby's head had not engaged. You also need to tell someone if your labour does not start within twenty-four hours because of the risk of infection, although you are probably better off going into labour naturally than being induced, providing that someone is keeping a close eye on you for possible signs of infection.

SHOW

'I waited in vain for a show, but if I had one, I never noticed it.'

A show is a sort of pinky browny discharge that occurs when the plug of mucus in the cervix comes away. It signifies that your womb is getting ready to do its thing; but don't hold your breath – it can come away as much as two weeks before delivery. On the other hand, it may occur just before labour starts or you may never even notice it – it's not something that is always instantly recognisable. As you may gather, it's not what might be called a reliable witness, and in the latter weeks of pregnancy, you don't need to tell anyone about it.

CONTRACTIONS

'It was like period pains at first and I remember thinking if this is all it is, I'll be fine. I soon changed my tune, I can tell you.'

'For about two weeks, my contractions would start, then stop. In the end, I ignored the real thing and we only just got to hospital in time.'

'I think I got some sort of record, I went in four times. In the end they kept me because I think they felt sorry for my husband.'

'I wish someone had told me that the "before" bit of labour could go on for so long. It was dreadful backache that I noticed first.'

'I had a bout of diarrhoea which I put down to the curry we'd had the night before, but that was the beginning really.'

'I had these cramps and I was hugging myself in bed, thinking "This is it, this is it".'

Your womb has in fact been practising contractions for some time before labour starts – the so-called Braxton Hicks contractions which you may experience as tightenings of your bulge. Labour is so highly individual that it is difficult to say exactly when it starts; each woman is different. It may start with waters breaking, but it is more likely to start with period-like cramps or backache. You may start to experience contractions which are as close as three minutes apart and may think, 'Oh my God, this is it, I'm one of those women who have babies in buses', having been told that three-minute contractions are where it's at. Very often, however, these contractions will fade and it is the intensity rather than the timing of the contractions that is of most importance. Basically you need to think about moving off when your contractions are very regular, and of increasing intensity, and either beginning to become overly uncomfortable, or if you feel that you will be happier being where you are booked to deliver. This latter notion may be heightened by other circumstances – like your distance from hospital, need to sort out other children, etc.

Many women mentioned a secret worry that they would not know when they were in labour. I suspect that this worry comes partly from stories like the one above, from friends or relatives who think they are in labour but who are firmly sent home as not being in labour, not once but several times. They might feel like twits, but it is actually very difficult even for professionals to be sure whether labour really has started, so it's not something you should feel intimidated about. Here's a rough guide: false labour pains tend to decrease when you get up and walk around, whereas if you are in labour, they increase. False labour pains never settle down to a proper rhythm; they may be regular for a bit, then all over the place. To confuse you, real labour pains do not, as some would have you believe, increase in strength and duration in a completely regular fashion, and you will find longer, stronger contractions quite often being interspersed with ones of less intensity. False labour pains tend not to increase in intensity over time.

Of course, just because you are having false labour pains does not mean that you are not in discomfort, or that this should be dismissed as insignificant because you are not yet actually in labour. On the contrary, it can be very demoralising and miserable. If you need pain relief, it's best to take paracetamol rather than aspirin which could temporarily adversely affect the baby's blood clotting system at this late stage. These rather irritating false labour pains may go on for any period between hours and days, and if it is the latter it can be very wearing. Try to carry on with life, but if you find that you are getting very tired, particularly if you are not able to sleep properly, you might try a homeopath as there are one or two homeopathic remedies, pulsatilla or caullophyllum (not suitable for self-diagnosis and administration), which in appropriate, properly supervised doses either send you on your way if you are ready, or stop the contractions. You also need to be warned about that other well known phenomenon – the hospital effect. There you are, having regular contractions; you get to hospital and everything stops for a couple of hours. It is very common, and normally they'll start off again once you have settled down and walked around a bit.

Eating in Labour

'There was my husband revving the car outside, and I was indoors stuffing scrambled eggs.'

Many women lose their appetite immediately prior to the onset of labour, and it may well be that you come into hospital not having eaten much in the previous twenty-four hours, with the prospect of eating nothing for the next twenty-four either, since most hospitals have a policy of no solid food during labour and only sips of clear fluids. There is a dilemma here. Starvation forces your body to mobilise fat as a source of energy, rather than glucose, producing an excess of ketones (substances chemically related to acetone – nail varnish remover). Your partner may notice the telltale smell of peardrops or a fruity smell on your breath, indicating excessive ketone formation (ketosis) and your urine (which will be tested routinely) may also indicate ketosis. Ketosis is to some extent a natural state (it develops after hard exercise) but can be more serious and can certainly make you sick, or feel nauseous. Ideally, you should eat (although you may not feel like much), preferably little and often, and you should certainly increase your intake of clear fluids. However, hospitals are concerned about acid aspiration (breathing acid vomit and food particles into your lungs should you require general anaesthesia) and so eating and drinking is often denied in favour of a glucose and salt drip which in itself could be the cause of minor glucose imbalance for the baby.

Acid aspiration is a real and serious problem but it is almost exclusively a problem of general anaesthesia, and probably in the very rare cases when it does occur it has much more to do with poor anaesthetic technique than what you've eaten. In fact, maternal deaths from acid aspiration rose rather than fell in the years following the introduction of strict dietary regimes during labour. In addition, the gut slows down during labour and thus there is no guarantee that even quite long periods without food will ensure that the stomach is empty. The reason why I am making this point at length is that unless a caesarean is a serious possibility, you are at such low risk that it is quite in order for you to have light snacks (such as crisp toast, biscuits, lightly cooked eggs, etc.) as well as clear fluids during labour as and when you need them, making you better equipped to cope with the intense physical demands of labour. You wouldn't expect to do something really strenuous in a half-starved state if you weren't pregnant, and the rationale behind starvation during labour is, as I hope I've made clear, less than convincing. Even if an emergency section has to be undertaken, you can be given antacids (industrial strength variations of Milk of Magnesia) to reduce the acidity of the stomach contents, or better still avoid the possibility of acid aspiration altogether by having an epidural. So, if you want scrambled eggs before you set off, have 'em.

It is an extraordinary feeling, that very beginning bit of labour. It's a mixture of anticipation and excitement. It's like stepping off a cliff. It's suddenly feeling ever so grown up but very small at the same time.

Knowing when to go into hospital is not easy and there are few hard and fast rules. If your waters have broken and twenty-four hours have elapsed with no labour pains, if your waters were green or smelly, if you have any bleeding, if you had a very fast previous delivery, these are all grounds for immediate admission. As for contractions, it is probably best to say that if they are getting very uncomfortable or are lasting about 45 seconds each, it is time to set off. And if you live miles from the hospital or have to negotiate heavy traffic, or have to make arrangements for other children, or simply don't feel right being at home still, you may want to set off before things get too far on. And, of course, you can always ring the hospital at any time for advice.

In Labour

DILATATION OF THE CERVIX

During the first part of labour – the latent phase – the cervix 'effaces', i.e. it becomes thinner, and then dilates. Dilatation is measured in centimetres. First-time labours generally progress at the rate of about 1 cm per hour. When the cervix has reached about 4 cm, a more active phase of labour begins, with the cervix continuing to dilate until it reaches about 8 cm.

During the transition phase, the cervix becomes fully dilated to 10 cm, and this is usually the most intense and painful part of labour. At the beginning of the second stage of labour, the mother has a desire to bear down with each contraction. As the baby moves down the birth canal, it rotates and then has to flex in order to get to the vaginal outlet which is upwards and forwards − sort of round the corner from where the baby is. The third stage of labour involves delivery of the placenta. If this is the theory, then there are infinite variations upon it. Although labour is presented as a smooth progression, with dilatation proceeding at a fixed rate, there are very often sudden accelerations, when there is a dramatic dilatation from say 6 cm to 10 cm in the space of as many minutes. At other times cervical dilatation comes to a grinding halt.

You would think, wouldn't you, that you would be able to feel whether your cervix was dilating or not. Actually, you have to rely completely on other people to tell you how far you have dilated. Dilatation is measured in the crudest of ways. Although there are fancy little cards, usually supplied by drug companies, showing series of circles with the appropriate measurements for comparison, the old-fashioned way is simply to note how many (gloved) fingers can be placed in the cervix.

Pain Relief

'Don't let anyone tell you it doesn't hurt. It was agony.'

'I psyched myself up so much about the pain, but when it came to it, it really wasn't that bad and I coped fine.'

'In the end if someone had said we're going to cut off your legs now and it'll all be over, I would have agreed.'

About a third of women will find labour pain much as they had expected it. About a third will find it more painful but a third will find it less painful than they had anticipated. There's no getting away from it. Labour hurts. I must have talked to thousands of women in my time, but can't remember more than half a dozen who claimed to have experienced little or no pain during labour. Interestingly, several of these were women who had had almost no warning of labour and who had had their babies very quickly, some within twenty minutes or so. Lest you should hate these women already, most of them found themselves confined to hospital for the latter part of subsequent pregnancies as these were precisely the women you read about in the papers, surprising cashiers at Tesco, astonishing sundry cab drivers and giving bobbies on the beat something to smile about after having successfully delivered a baby whilst on the day shift.

Before going into the various pain relief options, it's worth explaining the basis of pain. Very often you hear people say that they have a low pain threshold. In fact pain threshold is remarkably similar in all people, regardless of sexual, social or cultural differences, but these differences have a definite influence on an individual's perception of pain, so it is true to say that pain is personalised for each individual. Pain threshold increases in labour, partly due to the release of natural pain killers, endorphins, from the brain.

We often speak admiringly of people who put up with pain or who cope with it better than we think we could, but people develop various coping mechanisms to deal with it and it's highly likely that were you in the same situation, you would cope just as well. In some ways all the words we use to describe coping with pain, like being brave, being a hero, only compound the perception that somehow to be able to endure pain is noble and puts you on a higher moral plane. Nuts to that. There's no shame in saying that you need help to cope with pain — it's just a statement of physiological fact not an admission of failure. And there are no rewards handed out to those who do not need help.

Pain, or the possibility of pain, can induce fear in which anxiety borders on panic. Fatigue and sleep deprivation magnify pain. At the same time, pain stimuli that are particularly intense can, in effect, be ignored by the body. This is an important concept because it will help you understand why certain unlikely methods of pain relief, such as massage, can affect the perception of pain. Certain nerve cell groupings within the spinal cord and brain stem are thought to have the ability to modulate the pain impulse through a blocking mechanism. It's called the gate control theory. Local stimulation such as massage closes a hypothetical gate in the spinal cord, thus blocking pain signals from reaching the brain and perception of pain stimuli is also diminished. When a woman in labour performs activities that require concentration, such as particular types of breathing or counting, there is selective and directed brain activity which activates and closes the gating mechanism. At least this is the theory. It does work for some people, although only about 5 per cent of women rely on natural methods alone for pain relief throughout their labour.

Returning to my point about being flexible, you do not have to decide in advance what method of pain relief, if any, you are going to have. It's a sort of suck-it-and-see situation in which you try increasingly powerful methods of pain relief, as and when you need it. You might not need as much as you think or, alternatively, might need far more pain relief than you had envisaged. You might start off with massage and find that breathing and changing position is all you need. On the other hand, you might decide a couple of hours in that total pain relief in the form of an epidural is what you want. A frequent reason for dissatisfaction with labour is that women feel they have failed if, having planned a drug-free labour, pain gets on top of them and they accept pain relief. I think if this situation is one you get into, you have to be rational (or your partner has to be rational for you). Experiencing severe pain has many physiological effects, including lessening contractions and therefore prolonging labour. Severe maternal stress causes release of catecholamines which have been linked with fetal distress – so there are sound medical reasons for making sure that your pain is kept within acceptable limits.

There are advantages and disadvantages with all the methods I am going to outline; what you want to know is, how quickly they work (i.e. what's the time lag between administration and effect), and how effective they are. I also believe very firmly that you should have what you think is best for you, not what someone else believes is best for you. Pain relief is something that tends to throw up very strong opinions; you have to remember that they are just that, opinions based on personal experience, and not necessarily what is best for you. Do your own thing and be happy with whatever you choose.

CHANGE OF POSITION

There is a touch of the obvious about this, I know, but changing position during labour can dramatically affect pain because by changing position you alter the relationship between the baby, gravity, the pelvis and contractions. Moving about also helps improve circulation. Labouring women spontaneously adopt upright or squatting positions and walking may be especially effective. If you are having a lot of back pain, a hands–and–knees position may relieve it. It is up to you to shift around to try and find the position in which you feel most comfortable, using the bed, chair, cushions and even your partner as support. As the labour progresses, you will find that a once comfortable position has to be abandoned in favour of something else as the baby moves down the birth canal.

TOUCH AND MASSAGE

If you have a partner who is good at this, brilliant. There are several books which describe massage techniques for use in pregnancy and labour and you may find someone who is able to teach you and your partner these techniques prior to delivery. The massage can take many forms: it can involve stroking, vibration, kneading, deep circular pressure, continuous steady pressure and joint manipulation. It can involve the use of the fingertips, the whole hands or various devices which roll, vibrate or apply pressure. Although you will find that your perception of pain is heightened when the massage stops, intermittent massage is probably more effective, because if you carried on doing it continuously you would just adapt to it and lessen the effect. One word of warning – what you find intensely pleasurable in pregnancy may be downright irritating when you are in labour; your partner needs to be aware of this possibility and be prepared to change techniques or area of massage until he finds something that you find soothing. If you have bad backache, perhaps because you have a baby in an occipito-posterior position, counterpressure can be effective, in which your partner applies a strong pressure with either his fist or another object.

WATER

Given that hydrotherapy is very widely used in many other fields of medicine as a way of relieving pain, it is astonishing that it isn't more widely used in labour. Quite a few hospitals now have birthing pools, but it's not just immersion in water that is helpful. Directed showers are particularly effective and a combination of hot, then cold water may be very good for some women.

HOT AND COLD

There are lots of sound physiological reasons why heat and cold affect the perception of pain. Whilst the use of a hot-water bottle, blanket, compress or ice pack may simply be pain relief add-on rather than pain relief staples, they may have considerable comfort value.

DISTRACTION

At its most simple, distraction can involve going for a walk, getting out of the delivery room or watching something on television. We all know that concentrating hard on something can distract us from, for instance, period pain, so you might like to take something to do that requires mental concentration. A friend of mine, who had no pain relief for any of her four children, took the proofs of a book on women's health which we had been working on together. A number of chapters had been contributed by obstetricians and she was already annoyed by their lack of grammar and concern for rudiments of English, and incomprehensible jargon. So she took these chapters with her when she went into labour with her fourth baby and claimed that her frantic red pencilling got her through hours of labour without a thought as to pain.

MUSIC

Music has long been known to aid in pain relief. It may be that a favourite song or tune makes you feel good, or that the rhythm of it helps you with breathing or counting or helps your partner with massage strokes. It probably works best for those women for whom music is a particularly important part of their lives. You may prefer to play music on a tape recorder, or to listen through headphones, which has the added advantage of blocking out other sounds.

TENS

TENS stands for transcutaneous electrical nerve stimulation. It is a non-invasive form of pain relief that many women find effective, particularly if they use it from early labour onwards. For some women, however, it is totally ineffective; for others it is an irritation because it means wires and a bulky machine which get in the way if you want to walk about or have a pee. There are usually four electrode pads which, when placed on the skin (usually on your lower back), emit a variable electrical signal which is under your control, generated from a smallish box. You can choose to have a constant or a pulsing type of signal and there is a range of strengths. You get a sort of buzzing feeling and the TENS machine works on the gateway principle described earlier. You can hire a machine from the hospital in advance of your labour. Curiously, trials involving TENS usage have suggested that it increases the reported incidence of intense pain rather than decreasing it, whilst at the same time being favourably assessed as a method of pain control, which all goes to prove that there's nowt so queer as folk.

Pain Relief Using Drugs

PETHIDINE

Most people assume that pethidine, a powerful narcotic drug, will take pain away by anaesthetising you in some way. It actually isn't designed to do this. What it does is alter your perception of pain by acting as both a muscle relaxant and mood enhancer. Unfortunately these drugs have many unwanted side effects including dizziness, nausea and vomiting, as well as increasing the length of time undigested food remains in the gut. Pethidine also crosses the placenta and may have a marked effect on the baby, before and after delivery. After the birth, the baby may be very sleepy and unwilling to suck which can make establishing feeding difficult. These babies tend to be unsettled and difficult to comfort. Of greater concern, however, is a delay in breathing at birth which is caused by the baby's respiration being depressed by the action of the drug, especially if large or repeated doses have been used, or if the pethidine has been injected within the last few hours. If you are close to being fully dilated, you will be refused pethidine because of the likely effects on the baby. However, there is an antidote which can be injected into the baby's umbilical cord after birth if the baby is born more quickly than expected.

Many women describe being on pethidine as being 'floaty' or 'woozy', as if they'd been on nothing but neat gin all evening. You may feel confused and disorientated, just as you would if you were drunk, and unable to communicate properly. Alternatively you can feel on a 'high' with a sense of euphoria. An advantage of pethidine is that it can give you an opportunity to get some much needed sleep if you are very exhausted, because it makes you sleepy, but you have to set against this the experience of a sort of obstetric twilight zone in which you aren't quite all there as pethidine can cause a temporary amnesia. If pethidine is suggested, you might like to try a small dose at first and see how it makes you feel, because although you might be one of those people who feel great, you might also be one of those people on whom pethidine has no effect whatsoever or who feel disoerientated by it. Incidentally, dosage of pethidine is related to body weight which is why you may suddenly be asked how much you weigh.

Pethidine can be administered either intravenously (in which case the onset of effect is rapid, usually within 30 seconds, with maximum effect being reached in about 10 minutes and lasting up to 4 hours), or intramuscularly, in which case the onset is not as rapid (about 15 minutes). Some hospitals have self-administered IV systems and experience of these is that lower dosages are used and better pain relief obtained than that achieved through intramuscular injections. Curiously, the most appropriate time for pethidine may be after the birth, particularly if it has been long and very exhausting. You will find that you are so excited that sleep is almost impossible and a small dose may make all the difference to you feeling exhausted for days and unable to cope.

Some hospitals use tranquillisers and sedatives, particularly in early stages of labour, if they feel that it will help reduce anxiety and help you sleep. Barbiturates are not used in obstetrics, and sedatives tend to be either phenothiazine derivatives or benzodiazepines (e.g. Valium). They may also be used at the same time as narcotic agents as they have anti-emetic properties. Some, e.g. Valium, cause respiratory depression in babies. Frankly, a glass of something you fancy will probably do as well in early labour.

INHALATION DRUGS

'I hated the mask. It had a horrible rubbery smell and made me feel claustrophobic.'

'I found it really useful and it was just what I needed to help me through the last stages.'

'Once I sussed how to use it, it was pretty effective.'

These are pain-relieving agents that are inhaled. Entonox is a half-and-time mixture of oxygen and nitrous oxide (laughing gas) which is inhaled through either a mouthpiece (which many women prefer) or a rubber mask. The mask has a demand valve, which means that it is only released when you breathe in. You have to start using it before a contraction takes hold as the effect does not start for 10–20 seconds after you breathe in, reaching a peak after about a minute. It takes a bit of getting used to, as you need to breathe deeply but avoid the natural temptation to go on inhaling throughout the contraction. Instead a few breaths, no more than four or five at the start, with the mask being then put down, will allow the gas to reach a peak as your contraction peaks. If you carry on, you will feel so woozy that you will miss the next contraction. Like pethidine, Entonox numbs your sensation of pain rather than taking it away altogether. Like pethidine, gas and air may not work for everyone, and like pethidine it may make you feel sick or woozy. It is probably most effective in the earlier stages of labour (although prolonged use may make you feel very sick) and is not good at dealing with intense pain, particularly if your contractions start this way. It may make your mouth very dry, and you may need to suck a sponge between contractions, but it does have some advantages in that you can control how much you want to use and it may give you that little bit of extra pain relief you need if you are otherwise doing it on your own. The effects are very shortlived and it has a minimal effect on the baby – in fact, the extra oxygen may be helpful to the baby. If you are contemplating using Entonox, it would be a good idea to practise with it very early on in labour before the contractions have got out of hand, so that you get the hang of it for when you need it. Because the gas comes on a handy wheely thing and the rubber hose is long, quite a bit of mobility is possible.

EPIDURAL

'I was on the steps of the hospital waiting for my epidural.'

'I had complete pain relief and there was no comparison between my first labour (dreadful) and my second (wonderful).'

'Thank God for epidurals.'

'I'm glad I had an epidural in the end, because I don't think I could have coped any more with the pain, but my legs were numb for ages and I had to be manhandled by the staff afterwards because I couldn't walk.'

'It was bizarre watching the contractions on the monitor but not being able to feel them.'

'I had an epidural but I felt a bit cheated and a bit of a coward for having agreed to it.'

'I wish I hadn't had an epidural because it makes it all so clinical and next time I think I'll go for a natural delivery.'

'Nobody told me that you could have an epidural and it not work.'

'It didn't take effect straight away and I had twenty minutes of wishing I was dead.'

'Having had an epidural with my first baby, I wanted another one. When I had my second, I got into the hospital and my first words were 'epidural, please', only for the midwife to say that I was 9 cm dilated and there was hardly time to get me to the delivery room, let alone for me to have an epidural. Hannah was born forty minutes later.'

'Am I glad I had an epidural with my third. The others were bad enough at 9 lb and 9 lb 5 oz but Thomas was 10 lb 9 oz and trouble all the way.'

I think epidurals are one of those things that either you embrace wholeheartedly or that fill you with horror – there doesn't seem to be much middle ground. There is no doubt that an epidural medicalises labour, because once you have an epidural you are effectively grounded (unless you have the 'walking epidurals' offered by some hospitals, see page 245) because your legs are too numb to walk and because you are hooked up to monitors. Because an epidural causes the blood pressure to drop, you will have to have a drop on your arm to give you fluids and maintain your blood pressure at an adequate level. You will also have to have your blood pressure monitored every 15 minutes. You will have no sensation in the lower half of your body and it will therefore be necessary to put a fine narrow tube (catheter) into your bladder which will fill rapidly because of the fluids you are being infused with.

Setting up an epidural requires specialist skills and not all hospitals have twenty-four-hour obstetric anaesthesia, which may limit your access to epidurals. The anaesthetist will usually come and say hello when you book in, if you have requested an epidural. Quite often they will offer to set things up whilst you are still coping well with your contractions, leaving it up to you and your midwife when you actually start using it. This is probably a good idea because having not only to lie still for twenty minutes while the anaesthetist fiddles about, but then wait another twenty minutes or so while contractions are hitting you every couple of minutes, can be hell. It also gives you the option of not having an epidural if you find that you can cope with the pain after all. If you are too far dilated (say more than 8–9 cm) when you arrive, you will not be given an epidural, because second stage is imminent, and that is when you least want an epidural's ability to remove the urge to push.

The anaesthetic is injected into the space between your spine bones through a very thin tube. The tube is taped in place and a phial for administering the anaesthetic is strapped over your shoulder. Be warned, anaesthetists use serious needles for this job and although you can't see what's going on, your partner has a cracking view. If he is squeamish, you may prefer to have him round your side, so you can hold each other's hands. You may find that the pain relief isn't total, but is confined to just one side, or even that the pain relief is not very effective. Whatever you do don't sit there thinking 'is this how it's meant to be?' Ask for the anaesthetist to come back – sometimes resiting the catheter can sort things out. More anaesthetic can be administered when the effect begins to wear off, through the tube already in place.

There is a good deal of evidence that regular top-ups (every two hours) are more effective than demand top-ups.

Moderate to severe pain was only experienced by 14 per cent of women in a regular top-up arm of a trial, compared to 86 per cent of the demand group. I suspect that having to ask for a top-up is something women don't like to do until they are desperate – which isn't the object at all. Many units will try and avoid a top-up if you are at the transition stage, since epidurals take away your urge to push and it can be difficult to push the baby out if you are not quite sure where and how hard to push.

For this reason, forceps deliveries are more common in labours where epidurals are used. Babies often fail to rotate properly from an occipito-posterior position, meaning a higher incidence of rotational forcep use (Kiellands forceps). The second stage is also more likely to be prolonged. An epidural is a classic example of a medical procedure which begets other medical procedures – forceps, monitoring, drips, etc. – so in some ways having an epidural is like getting on to a merry-go-round which you can't get off. You should therefore be aware what it involves before you decide to have one.

'Walking epidurals' were originally developed at Queen Charlotte's Hospital in London because anaesthetists were aware that women wanted to lose the pain, not to feel nothing. At first they tried diluting the dose of anaesthetic (conventionally bupivacaine) but this didn't work, so they added another painkilling drug, fentanyl, which enhances the effect of bupivacaine. Combinations of this were injected into the extradural space, but women still suffered from a total block after a couple of hours, so a different approach was adopted, in which a very fine needle is put into the spinal fluid space, and an initial combination dose given, followed with top-ups in the epidural space. This seems to work a treat and in fact was the subject of one of my *Tomorrow's World* films. It seems a complete contradiction in terms, but the lady I accompanied throughout her labour continued to have full feeling in her legs and to be able to walk around, whilst not feeling her contractions. She was monitored by telemetry (radio tracking – like you use to track polar bears or other animals in the wild) and had a 'giving set' which enabled her to top up her dose herself. To me there were many advantages of this system – walking helped counteract the slowing effect of labour that conventional epidurals tend to have, and the giving set meant that women could deal sensitively with their own pain rather than arguing with a midwife about how much pain they were in.

As one of our survey respondents remarked, it is rather a surreal experience to know that you are having contractions, because you are seeing them on a monitor, but not to experience them. For women having epidurals, labour is a pretty leisurely affair and you and your partner will probably need something to do, like a game to play, to kill the time. If instrumental deliveries are necessary, the epidural may have to be topped up right at the end. Although the delivery will be pain free, it does mean that you have another couple of hours or so of not having your legs work properly, which may mean having to be lifted back to the ward. This can be rather demeaning because you are a completely helpless dead weight. If you think there is a possibility that you might have to have a caesarean, an epidural is a very good choice of pain relief because, if a section turns out to be necessary, it can simply be topped up. For some women, epidurals cause long-term backache. However, the post-birth period is a time when many women experience backache for the first time, their backs having been put out of alignment by pregnancy and then abused by constant lifting of small heavy objects (to wit, babies) in impossibly awkward situations (from baths, cots and the back of cars) and I am not personally convinced that epidurals deserve all the blame.

There are other potential side effects. Paralysis has sometimes been cited and not surprisingly frightens most women witless. In a review of over 27,000 women having epidurals, only 9 had serious side effects and in only 3 of these cases was there serious concern for the health of the women. This review was in 1985 and there is now far greater experience of epidurals, so I personally wouldn't let this even cross your mind. Rather more likely is a severe headache, resulting from a dural tap (where the dura mater has been punctured and cerebrospinal fluid leaks out) which may mean having to lie flat for a couple of days after delivery. If the problem continues, it is fairly easily rectified with an epidural blood patch – some of your own blood injected into the epidural space literally to patch the hole.

So there you have the whole gamut of pain relief from partial to total. Pain in labour is inevitable but it is not quite the same as any other type of pain in that it has a purpose and it is limited in its duration. Many women are prepared to tolerate more pain than they perhaps might in any other situation, but what they are not prepared to do is to have pain overwhelm them. Read all of this very carefully and, at the risk of repeating myself, keep an open mind.

Monitoring

Women seem to be divided on the question of monitoring. Some like the reassurance that electronic monitoring can provide. Others resent its intrusion. The problem is that a baby consumes oxygen at twice the rate of an adult per unit weight and has an oxygen reserve which is only enough to meet its metabolic needs for 1–2 minutes. Bloodflow to the baby is temporarily interrupted during a contraction. A normal baby can withstand the stress of labour without suffering from lack of oxygen (hypoxia) because sufficient oxygen exchange goes on between contractions. But if a baby's oxygen supply is a bit dodgy – because, for instance, you are having closely spaced, lengthy contractions – the baby will become hypoxic (lacking in oxygen). There are two immediate consequences of this. The first is that various receptors strategically placed around the baby's body will send out signals which influence the baby's heartbeat, giving rise to contraction-related heart rate changes. The second is that the baby is forced into anaerobic metabolism – that is, forced to do some body work without oxygen. You have a similar and very familiar process in your body when you run fast. There is a sudden need for energy in your muscle, which would normally be obtained from glucose. But your muscle needs oxygen to convert glucose to energy and the demand for energy may outstrip the available oxygen supply. So the body tries to do the job without oxygen (anaerobically) which is possible, but one of the by-products is lactic acid which if it isn't cleared away fast enough gives you cramp. Now the baby also produces lactic acid but it doesn't cause cramp. Instead, the baby's blood becomes acidic.

Like your body, the baby's body is engaged in ceaseless activity which maintains the blood at a constant pH (pH is a measure of how alkaline or acid something is) no matter what's going on in the body. If the pH of the blood falls below 7.25 it indicates that however hard the baby is trying to keep its blood acidity stable, it is fighting a losing battle and is in distress. I'm sorry to make this such a lengthy explanation but I find that the words hypoxia and acidosis are very often bandied about but very rarely adequately explained, which can leave you feeling very confused. Sampling the baby's blood pH – you may also hear the phrase 'assessing the acid base balance', which amounts to much the same thing – usually via a scalp clip monitor can therefore give very important information. You might think that measuring the baby's blood oxygen level would be a better way of telling whether the baby was suffering from lack of oxygen, but a curious bit of chemistry called the Bohr effect occurs when the blood becomes acidic, meaning that the measured oxygen level will only fall slightly below normal levels, even though the baby may be very severely lacking in oxygen.

Having instructed you in chemistry, here's a small lesson on fetal heart rate patterns. The problem here is that the baby's heart rate can go wandering all over the place, even though its blood chemistry is fine and the baby has a good Apgar score at birth. In fact up to 80 per cent of abnormal fetal heart rate (FHR) patterns come from babies that are quite healthy, so FHR monitoring during labour can only ever be a screening process, not a diagnostic technique.

The abnormal patterns are decelerations (when the FHR slows down) and accelerations. Frequent dips in FHR can be caused by something as simple as the mother's position – and if you roll over on to your side, thereby relieving pressure on the cord by the baby, and taking the weight of the heavy womb off the vessel returning blood to your heart, and thence your placenta, the problem may disappear. If these so-called variable decelerations are seen when an oxytocin drip is being used, the drip will be discontinued as it is causing overly strong and too closely spaced contractions for the baby to cope effectively. Breathing oxygen may help. If an abnormal FHR persists despite these measures, scalp pH sampling is indicated, with measurements noted at frequent intervals. This is a far more effective measure of fetal distress, as I have indicated, and predicts fetal outcome 82 per cent of the time, with a false negative rate of about 10 per cent.

About 50 per cent of fetal distress occurs in labours known to be high risk. About 50 per cent occurs in labours following perfectly normal pregnancies. So does this mean that electronic monitoring should be used in all labours? For a while, in the late seventies and eighties, there was great enthusiasm for universal electronic monitoring which everyone assumed would reduce the number of babies damaged as a result of distress during labour. But a large number of trials, including a particularly well designed one in Dublin, showed that there was no decrease in the rate of fetal death in the womb, nor was there a decrease in the number of babies born with neurological abnormalities (although there was a decrease in the number of babies who had seizures). These studies confirmed what had been suspected for some time, which is that most brain damage in newborn babies is caused not by events in labour but by events during pregnancy, and could not therefore be prevented by current concepts in electronic monitoring.

So where does this leave you? The consensus of opinion in America is that high risk women should have continuous fetal monitoring or auscultation (listening with a fetal stethoscope or with an electronic device) every 15 minutes during the first stage and every 5 minutes in the second stage of labour. For low risk women, auscultation every 30 minutes in the first stage and every 15 minutes in the second stage is recommended. The policy in Britain varies from hospital to hospital, but many undertake what is known as strip monitoring, in which you will be hooked up for monitoring on admission. The idea behind this is that if there are any problems, they may be evident early on and therefore prompt continuous monitoring.

Equipment varies across the country, but most monitoring machines involve wearing a rather uncomfortable belt, which measures both the strength of your contractions and the FHR. Some hospitals use telemetric monitoring, which means that you can walk around. Telemetry does have some problems, however. A unit in the West Country noticed the traces from one woman going completely haywire. They rushed to find her, expecting heaven knows what, only to discover that she was outside, watching an air-sea rescue helicopter coming in to land. The strange FHR turned out to be interference from the helicopter's electronics. The moral is obviously to stay away from helicopters during labour if you can. If you have raised blood pressure, are diabetic or have other chronic disease, or if you have had previous problems during labour, you must expect to be monitored continuously.

Birth

Some hospitals have an arbitrary upper time limit on the second stage – for instance, that you may not push for more than an hour without intervention. This is because some obstetricians consider that sustained pushing results in damage to the perineal floor and consequently to a greater incidence of incontinence. This is hotly contested and many people take the view that while both mother and baby's vital signs are good, the second stage should last as long as it takes. Monitoring the baby's heartbeat can become very difficult during this stage of labour, mainly because the baby is deep in the pelvis. It is at this moment that you may be asked if a clip monitor can be attached to your baby's scalp and, since the information that such monitoring provides has a high degree of accuracy, it is probably a wise move, although continuous monitoring at this stage is not regarded as necessary except where circumstances warrant it.

When the baby is delivered and the cord cut, and perhaps

after the baby's airways have been suctioned (not policy in all hospitals), the baby will be placed on you, as is – i.e. covered in vernix, the whitish greasy covering babies have in the womb, and blood – for you to cuddle. Skin-to-skin contact like this is blissful – and important to the baby, whose temperature control mechanisms are not yet perfected and who needs the warmth of your body. The baby will have to be removed briefly to be weighed, tagged, scored (babies get marks out of ten, their Apgar score, dependent on a whole series of variables) and examined and to have an injection of vitamin K, but this is usually very brief and not done immediately. The baby is also likely to be wiped at this stage and wrapped. You may want to put the baby to the breast for a nuzzle. Medical staff are usually very aware of the need for all three of you to be together alone, and, having sorted out your immediate needs, will beat a swift retreat.

At this point, many women experience an overwhelming sense of joy and intense closeness with their partner. But if this is not how you feel, don't be alarmed. If you have had a difficult birth, you may be so dazed, exhausted and out of it that feelings will seem a luxury. Even if you haven't had a difficult delivery, it may take time for you to grow accustomed to your baby and to love her. Falling in love with your baby on her arrival and not doing so until much, perhaps even a couple of months, later, are both normal reactions. Doing so later doesn't mean that you are not maternal, simply that it didn't hit you this way – nothing more. Love takes many different forms and arrives in different ways, but how it happens is no indicator as to its eventual quality.

'Third stage, what third stage?'

'I had no idea what they were up to down there. I knew

they had lights and my feet were in stirrups but frankly I couldn't have cared less, all I could see was my baby.'

'I was scared about having an episiotomy but in the end, my baby was 10 lbs 3 ozs and I didn't have any option.'

'My husband stood there when I had my last baby (my fourth) saying "sew her up tight, doc, she'll be like the Ganges now." '

'Pregnancy and birth were fine but the episiotomy I had wrecked the next six months of my life.'

In certain circumstances, at delivery, an episiotomy – a deliberate cut of the perineum – is essential in order to avoid extensive tearing, when there is a big baby or an abnormal presentation or a medical procedure requiring forceps, etc. Over two-thirds of women in developed countries will have some tearing of the perineum during delivery requiring stitches. Some midwives are particularly good at 'guarding the perineum', holding their hands against the perineum during contractions, thus supporting the tissues enough to reduce trauma, and others advocate massaging the perineum with oil. Both practices are logical, although not scientifically evaluated. Of certain benefit is the role of the midwife during crowning (when the baby's head appears). In a nutshell, if you push your baby out with great speed and force, extensive tearing is likely, which is why the midwife will encourage you to pant, not to push, at a time when all you want to do is push. She is aiming for a controlled delivery of the baby, not a demonstration that she has the skills of an American quarterback in being able to dive and catch a slippery object at speed. And incidentally, to answer several unvoiced concerns from the survey, no, they won't fail to catch the baby – the whole point, as I said, is a controlled delivery.

For many years there has been over-liberal use of episiotomy, which remains the most common cause of perineal damage and which is carried out on between 50 to 90 per cent of women during a first delivery. The theory behind such extensive use is that it prevents damage to the anal sphincter and rectal area (third and fourth degree tears), avoids damage to the muscles of the pelvic floor, prevents trauma to the baby's head and, in having straight rather than ragged edges to sew up, makes repair easier and more effective. Long-term studies have failed to prove any of the above, although the role of episiotomy in preventing long-term incontinence remains a controversial issue. You may prefer to state in your birth plan, if your hospital has these, that you would prefer not to have an episiotomy unless absolutely necessary.

Another issue is, who should do the stitching when you have a tear or an episiotomy? There is a tendency in some hospitals for it to be done by the most junior member of the medical staff available as this is regarded as 'good practice' – where this phrase means not the more reassuring 'best practice' but 'here's a good way to learn skills on the job'.

It can be alarming to be faced with a green senior house officer, whose last needlework was a cross stitch mother's day gift made in primary school. In all honesty, however, insisting that you are only stitched by someone senior means that experience, and thus developing skills, are denied to women on a wider scale; yet you still want someone to do it well. A quick word to the midwife will usually reassure you as to the competency of your stitcher, but if you need extensive stitching rather than just a running repair, then I would insist on someone senior to do it. You will be placed in lithotomy stirrups, usually whilst you cuddle your baby, and using a good light source, plus additional anaesthesia if required, you will be stitched once the placenta has been delivered. If you have had a drug free labour, you will need pain relief (usually a local injection) while you are stitched. These injections usually take a little while to work, and if someone is being over-enthusiastic about getting on with it before you are numb, tell them, don't suffer in silence. Some women use gas and air at this point, although I personally think that you are better concentrating on your baby, rather than having to grit your teeth after a long exhausting labour.

In order to prevent post-partum haemmorhage (a danger-ous emergency), virtually all hospitals in the UK give an injection of Syntometrine (a combination of two drugs, syntocinon and ergometrine) to help deliver the placenta. This regime of drugs results in an important reduction in the risk of haemorrhage of between 30–40 per cent. Having a Syntometrine injection is not, however, a guarantee that you will not haemorrhage. It does cause nausea and vomiting in some women, as well as headache, and there is a small question mark about whether it causes a rise in blood pressure. So why not adopt the natural approach? A recent trial compared active management of the third stage of labour (giving syntometrine or similar drugs, clamping the cord early and cord traction – pulling the cord to bring the placenta out) with a 'natural' physiological approach, in which no drugs were given, the cord was clamped after delivery and the placenta was delivered by the mother, rather than by cord traction. The women with the active regime had less blood loss, fewer blood transfusions, shorter third stages, but were more likely to be sick.

You might think that you could mix and match, as it were – have pain relief, perhaps an epidural in the first stage, allow it to wear off, and then have a totally natural third stage. However, it's not like this. The effects of the epidural or of other pain relief prevent the third stage from being absolutely straightforward, so if you want to avoid Syntometrine and 'active management' of the third stage, it is only appropriate if you have had a completely natural labour. If you have rhesus negative blood, you will not have the cord clamped because it increases the risk of the baby's blood cells getting in to your blood and thereby potentially affecting subsequent pregnancies.

'I insisted on not having a Syntometrine injection. I then passed out because I haemorrhaged so badly.'

Sometimes the womb is not the source of the bleeding. Injuries to some part of the birth canal, either those which arise spontaneously during labour or those that are caused by a procedure are the problem. Tears to tissues at the outlet of the birth canal and episiotomies can bleed ferociously, although the blood loss can be easily controlled by pressure. Tears in the upper vagina or neck of the womb need to be inspected in an operating theatre, usually under general anaesthesia, although if you have had an epidural this may be adequate. Again, pressure will stop the bleeding, following which the wound can be stitched. These stitches are the dissolvable type and will not need removal after healing is completed.

FAST LABOUR

Although a fast labour sounds like every girl's dream come true, it can in fact be rather frightening. Contractions come thick and fast and you may feel completely overwhelmed. Very often there is no time to sort out an epidural so you may have to rely on gas and air, even though the contractions may be very painful. It is easy to panic in this situation, but the best thing to do is to get down on all fours or to squat whilst leaning forward as this will take some of the pressure off your cervix and slow things down a tad, so you at least get a chance to get your breath back.

SLOW LABOUR

Slow labours can be very tedious indeed. They can come to a grinding halt at different phases. Normally the latent phase of labour – the early part of the first stage – lasts anything up to twenty hours in first time mothers. If it lasts longer than this, it can be due to several causes. The first is that the woman isn't really in labour at all but in false labour which is pretty miserable. The second is that inappropriate use of sedatives or heavy analgesia too early in labour has slowed things down, and if this is the case labour will usually get going of its own accord when the effect of the drugs has worn off. Finally, it could be that the womb is either contracting too much, but being ineffective (in which case it needs to be rested using drugs), or contracting too little (in which case an oxytocin infusion will sort it out). In general, problems with the latent phase of labour can usually be resolved and the remainder of labour proceed normally.

It is difficult to cope with prolonged labour of this sort and walking around, frequent changes of scenery, or having a relaxed, warm bath will help you mentally as well as physically. You might also try a discreet bit of nipple twiddling; this stimulates the production of oxytocin. Trouble is, you'd probably need to do it for so long that it would end up being a bit of a duty rather than a pleasure. *Courage, mes braves.*

Sometimes labour comes to a halt during the active phrase, either because the cervix is stubbornly refusing to dilate any further for a couple of hours (an arrest of dilatation) or because the baby is refusing to come down any further (an arrest of descent). Again there can be a number of causes: either the baby is presenting awkwardly (i.e. not in the conventional manner) or perhaps there could be cephalo-pelvic disproportion, that is, the baby's head is too big or you are too small for it to be able to descend any further. If the cause is neither of these things, then labour may start again with an oxytocin infusion. If there is what is called a 'protraction' – in other words, things slow down but they don't stop altogether, oxytocin won't do any good and it is better to be patient and let things take their course naturally. This is difficult advice to take when you are the one it is happening to, and sensible pain relief, lots of support from your partner and frequent small snacks and drinks are essential if you are not to become exhausted. Make sure that you empty your bladder every hour as a full bladder can also slow things down.

BIG BABIES

Very often in clinic, or even when you are out and about, people will make remarks about your size, such as, 'you've got a big one there.' Whilst you may be able to ignore your mother-in-law or your next door neighbour, it can be rather more disquieting when the prophet of doom is a midwife or doctor. Very often these remarks are just small talk, and you should know that it is actually very difficult to assess the eventual weight and size of your baby accurately. And even if the weight is accurate, whether labour will be easy or difficult will depend on the shape of your pelvis and the baby's position within it, which it is even more difficult to be accurate about. My obstetrician managed to convince me that I was carrying something the size of a mastodon, only for me to give birth to a baby who was bang on the British male baby average weight of 3,333 g (7 lb 5 oz). If you have a very tall or big partner, whilst you are on the petite side, you may also be concerned, but although height and weight are genetically determined (and therefore inherited from both mother and father), the controlling factor in pregnancy is the size of the mother's womb. It's once they are out that they start to shoot up. The exception is diabetic pregnancy where macrosomia (a baby that is too big) is common, especially when the mother's diabetes is not well controlled. These pregnancies are usually induced several weeks before term if the size of the baby is causing concern.

Big babies can cause problems during labour, extending the length of the labour and also resulting in a higher incidence of deliveries by forceps although, as I have indicated, this is by no means always the case, as so many other factors, such as the size of the pelvis and position of the baby come into play. Alternatively labour may proceed well until it comes to delivering the shoulders, when things may get difficult, but usually this problem is resolved without too much drama.

BREECH BABIES

Breech babies sit upright in the womb, with their head underneath your ribs and their bottom firmly sitting on your cervix. There are several different types of breech, depending on whether the baby is curled up (complete), has its legs extended upwards (incomplete), or has one foot dangling beneath it (footling). In the past attempts have been made to turn breech babies by manipulating the abdomen, using a muscle relaxant after 37 weeks. Some claim as much as a 75 per cent success rate with this, but often the babies stubbornly return to their previous comfy spot. There are various methods to help turn a breech baby, such as adopting a head–to–knees position every day.

Because of their peculiar position, labour may be longer

and more tiring for the mother, but the main problem comes with the actual delivery when the head has to be delivered as quickly as possible after the rest of the body. Hospitals differ widely in their policies on breech deliveries and each case has to be treated individually. Some hospitals automatically deliver breech babies by caesarean; others are more relaxed. Certainly you should go into a breech delivery prepared that a caesarean section might be necessary, although it is entirely possible that you will deliver spontaneously. Perinatal mortality rates for breech babies are four times higher than those for normally positioned babies. However, if strict criteria are adopted about which breech babies are suitable for vaginal and which for caesarean section (for instance that the baby is of normal size, and the mother's pelvis adequate), perinatal mortality rates for breech babies delivered vaginally do not differ significantly from those delivered by caesarean.

DELIVERIES WITH FORCEPS OR VACUUM EXTRACTOR

In the past, it used to be that all babies in some hospitals were delivered using forceps. In this way, trainee obstetricians built up a vast amount of experience and were very effective at using forceps properly as a result. There are lots of different sorts of forceps: some are what might be called 'lift-out jobs', just giving that extra bit of help to a woman finding it hard to expel the baby, whilst others are specially designed not only to take the baby out from high in the pelvic cavity but to turn it as well (so called rotational forceps, of which the best known type are called Kiellands forceps). They look a bit like exotic salad servers, except that they come in two bits which slot together after having been put on either side of the baby's head. A vacuum extractor or ventouse does much the same job as forceps. Basically it is a suction cap which is attached to the baby's head. A vacuum is created in the cap which is used to help pull the baby out. In trials, a vacuum extractor comes out best, being less invasive, with less damage to the mother, but I've always suspected that this is possibly because it is easier to become accomplished with this technique than it is with forceps. However, if forceps are what you have always used, then that's what you are better at – it is very much the skill of the operator that counts.

For forceps deliveries in particular, adequate pain relief is essential and either a spinal block or pudendal block (effective forms of local anaesthetic) may be used. Babies tend to have red marks on their heads but these very quickly fade. You will need to be in the lithotomy position (with your legs up in stirrups) and may have to have an episiotomy with forceps. If you think this sounds very alarming, take heart; my second baby was wedged fast in an occipito-posterior position (looking the wrong way – something he has continued to do since birth) and I emerged from a Kiellands forceps delivery with not a scratch on me, nor on Ellis either, so mashed bits and pieces are certainly not inevitable with forceps, although you will feel pretty bruised.

Labour Niggles

The foregoing shows the big picture of labour, but in the survey we found that many of you worried too about seemingly minor things. Here are some of those worries, many of them, it appeared, not articulated at the time, that you told us about in confidence in the survey returns.

'My husband passed out cold when I cut my finger and I don't think he'll cope with all that blood at the birth.'

'I was more worried about Tom fainting in the delivery suite than I was about the labour.'

'Will I see much blood? That's the thing that worries me most.'

There is no hiding that there can be quite a bit of blood around as the baby is delivered but if you are a bit iffy about blood, as many people are, don't worry; you won't ever be able to see much, simply because you are at the wrong end of the proceedings. Similarly, if your partner is not sure about blood, say that you want him up with you, not down the business end, and for heaven's sake tell your carers that you (or he) are squeamish, before someone in a fit of enthusiasm shows you the placenta in all its glory. Actually, it's my experience that even though there is a bit of gore about, it will pass unnoticed because your eyes see nothing except your baby. Similarly, if you (or your partner) are worried by needles, tell someone and have it put on your notes. Quite a number of alarmingly sized needles are used during labour, especially if you are having an epidural (don't worry – only the tip of the needle goes in) and it may be better if your carer asks you to look away for a bit. But they will only know to do that if you've told them about your needle concerns in advance.

'I was worried I'd soil myself in labour.'

'What if I did a poo during birth?'

'I was really embarrassed about shitting myself.'

Variations on this theme were the single most common 'worry I never told anyone about' in our survey. The gut slows right down during labour, but pressure of the presenting part and exertion can push any stool present in the anal canal out. This is pretty common and your carers will certainly not be in the least bit embarrassed about it. They are likely to clear any mess away very discreetly and you may not even be aware that it has happened. Often, the gut has slowed to such a degree that there aren't any stools present, although when the baby is deep in the pelvis it can feel as though you need to defecate, even though there is no stool there when you come to bear down. So, it doesn't always happen and even if it does, it really isn't a big deal – just part of reproductive life's rich pageant – and perfectly normal. If you are very concerned about this, you might be tempted to ask for an enema. Apart from being a horrible experience, all an enema does is clear one part of your bowel – simply allowing stools from higher up the gut to occupy the vacated space – so there is no guarantee that it will have the desired effect. Talk this over with your carers and you will very soon be reassured.

'I was worried about being seen naked.'

'The thought of complete strangers seeing the most intimate parts of my body didn't worry me, but my husband got in a right state about it.'

'Couldn't I be covered up with a blanket or something?'

A woman once told me that her husband regarded her body as a temple. They both felt strongly that no one else should violate her temple but she was now pregnant and this was proving something of a problem. Was it possible for the obstetrician to stand outside the labour room door and shout instructions to her husband so that he could perform any intimate moves necessary during the birth of their baby? Truly. This might be an extreme point of view, nevertheless privacy and dignity are essential to your wellbeing. It also helps you feel less intimidated by medical procedures if you are at least semi-clothed, which is why you might be well advised to wear your own clothes in labour, rather than hospital gowns which never, but never, seem to come equipped with the cords that are supposed to tie them modestly at the back. You may feel very shy about your naked body being seen by other people and may be even more concerned about so many people seeing such intimate parts of you. Your carers are likely to be much less cavalier than they were in the past about privacy and many hospitals strive to be scrupulous about knocking before entering your delivery room, asking you if you mind other people coming in, making sure you are covered if you want to be, etc. However, it has to be said that once they are in established labour, and even more so when they are pushing, most women couldn't care less whether three divisions of the Grenadier Guards marched through the room. All you can think about is concentrating on those contractions and getting that baby out. Somehow sexuality goes out of the window.

'My greatest worry was whether I'd cope.'

'I'm not very brave and my greatest fear is not to be able to cope with it all.'

Concerns about 'coping' during labour were immensely common, with nearly a quarter of our survey respondents saying that it was something they were very worried about. But only a little over half of these women found coping a problem with hindsight. I think it is important that you rationalise what you mean by 'not coping'. For most women it means, and I am using a selection of the phrases that women themselves used: wimping out; making a complete fool of myself; breaking down; being out of control; hysteria; screaming and shrieking, and even packing my bags and leaving. Tricky one that when you are in the middle of labour. All these are very real fears and all, in some way or another, relate directly to a loss of self-esteem when rising pain levels induce a sense of fear and panic which you feel will in some way demean you in the eyes of those with you. We all fear humiliation; it is an immensely understandable, indeed universal human fear and the fear is amplified during labour simply because there is no turning back. It's too late to decide that you'd rather not have a baby and go home as that one phrase above suggests but it's the one thought that probably has come to all of us during labour – why on earth did I think this was a good idea?

Stop right here. The first thing to say is that, rather like the fears about defecating in labour, there isn't anything that midwives haven't seen before and nothing that you do or say during labour will not have been done or said by a million other women before you. Health professionals are not secret spies handing out points for extra bravery in the face of pain or drama. They are trained professionals who do the job because they have a genuine concern for the women in their care. They are there to help you and will not think the worse of you, or refuse to help or not support you, simply because *you* think you are being a fool. Rely on their expertise to get you through labour. Realise that pain relief is only ever a few minutes away should you need it, and that labour, though it might seem like it, doesn't go on for ever.

> '*I thought my partner would find it very difficult. In the end I told him not to come and Mum came instead and I think it was better all round.*'

'Dave said he didn't want to be there all along and I was very disappointed. But at the last moment, I think he felt so sorry for me and came in. The nurses couldn't have got him out with a bomb after that.'

'I don't know how I would have managed without my husband.'

'I did it without him being there and although he's wonderful with the baby, I still feel let down and hurt. He has always been a bit iffy about anything medical but I thought that he should have been able to put that behind him for the sake of me and the baby.'

'He fainted when the anaesthetist came in the room. He hadn't even done anything.'

For some couples nothing, but nothing, would persuade the man not to be there for his baby's birth. For other couples, cultural considerations may decide the choice of birth partner. However, for a few couples, there is disappointment and conflict because the male partner feels genuinely uncomfortable about being present, either because he believes it to be 'a woman's thing' or because he is not sure about his own ability to cope. There are women in this situation who feel that their partners may be more of a liability than a support, and make plans for another birth partner right from the beginning, but I suspect that these women are in the minority, the others feeling a sense of deep hurt which may or may not be articulated.

It's difficult to know how to resolve these problems. Perhaps you could involve your partner in classes, get him to talk it over with other men; but sometimes this approach serves only to compound their worries. Another tack may be to suggest that your partner comes in with you with the provision that he is free to bale out when or if he becomes uncomfortable. One advantage of this approach is that your partner will find out that what he can do is genuinely helpful. Another is that the experience may be infinitely less traumatic than he fears. A friend of mine fell very much in the 'woman's work' category and was not planning to be present at the birth. I told him that if anything were to go wrong, he would never be able to forgive himself for not having been there to help. I also told him that it would be one of the great moments of his life. It was the former that persuaded but the latter that happened to him – as I knew it would.

Do not, however, expect all men to fall in love instantly with their babies at their birth. It's a bit like falling in love with a partner – very few experience love at first sight (in fact most of us are extremely suspicious that such a thing exists) and for most it takes time. Sometimes the baby is something to be admired, but well down the list of priorities after a long and difficult labour. After all, your man chose you, not the baby, and seeing you go through it for hours without being able to do anything other than offer moral support may be an experience that ends with an overwhelming and very under-standable sense of relief that it is all over for you, rather than joy about the baby.

All hospitals will allow you to have one or more birthing companions with you. Some hospitals will allow children into the delivery room. Others prefer not, although for some women, taken by surprise in the wee small hours, accompany-ing children are a practical necessity.

'My language; talk about effing and blinding.'

'I remember throwing something at my husband at one stage and he was only trying to help, too.'

There are often veiled references in books to what is the labour equivalent of road rage. There will usually be a phrase which reads along the lines of 'women may become irritable at this stage [usually transition, when labour begins to change gear]'. I don't think that women's partners are sufficiently prepared for what may actually happen. Extreme anger may be directed towards the partner (it's all your fault for getting me into this mess), usually involving any amount of blue language and even violence. There may be periods when whatever your partner does to help will not find favour, being rejected in the most ungrateful and dismissive manner. In short, you will turn into a complete cow. It's quite beyond your control of course and for a while your partner may be confused and even upset. He needs to remain calm and understanding, because in the end his support is a crucial part of your defence against pain and exhaustion.

'I was haunted by cramp, it was almost worse than the labour pain.'

'It was just as well I'd decided not to have an epidural. I kept getting cramp and leapt off the bed vertically several times.'

For some reason, perhaps because you tend to point your toes when in pain, cramp can be a serious problem in labour, particularly in the calves. One might speculate that cramp occurs because of the extremely rapid depletion of calcium by the uterine muscles (calcium is essential to muscle contraction) during labour, and you might consider taking Dolomite or other calcium tablets prior to labour, but I am not convinced that there is any real science behind this. Massage is good, as is counter-stretching (pulling your foot up towards you, for instance). You may find a pair of woolly socks helpful.

*'After I'd had the baby, I got the shakes – the only time
that I can remember having shakes like that was when I
was little and I'd just been sick.'*

*'I remember trembling violently early in labour. My
husband was very concerned because he thought I'd
lost it altogether, but I think it was excitement.'*

*'Why did no one ever tell me that I would shake like a
leaf throughout labour?'*

It is not at all uncommon for women to have an attack of the
shakes at some time during labour. Whilst shakes are often
connected with cold, this is rarely the cause in labour. As one
woman suggested, excitement has something to do with it, as
does tension and shock. It is unusual for the shakes to last long.
A bit of cosseting, by which I mean your partner helping you
to a comfy supported position, having something sweet to eat
(this may be the moment to indulge in a bit of chocolate) and
some slow breathing will probably do the trick.

*'Nobody ever told me that you could be sick all through
labour.'*

*'I had a cup of tea immediately after the baby was born.
It was bliss but I was then violently sick which spoiled it
all a bit.'*

'I felt sick all the time.'

Again, nausea and vomiting are very frequent complaints in
labour. The causes as you might imagine are many and various.
Vomiting at the beginning of labour, as with diarrhoea, may
simply be the body's way of clearing the system. Hormonal
changes, tension, fear, side effects of drugs (especially

pethidine), low blood sugar, ketosis (see page 219) can all be culprits. It is also incredibly common for women to want a cup of tea immediately after delivery, and then just as common to throw up. Being sick can be very unpleasant at the best of times, let alone in labour. You may find frequent sips of water and small amounts of food like boiled sweets or dry biscuits are helpful. Relaxing between contractions may also help. If it is unbearable, there are some anti-emetic drugs available.

> 'The funniest thing in labour was when I tried to use the toilet. I was desperate to go, but couldn't make anything happen. The midwife came and turned the taps on in the toilet, but that didn't work, the doctor suggested running my wrists under cold water, but it was the consultant poking his head around the door saying how about a catheter that did it in the end.'

During labour it becomes difficult to urinate spontaneously, partly because of the pressure of the baby's head on the bladder. It is nevertheless important that you empty your bladder regularly as otherwise it may become damaged by being over-distended and become a source of problems, specifically infection, after the birth. A full bladder may also slow down labour. If you can't manage a trip to the loo, you will be offered a bedpan which may make matters even worse, as in my experience your ability to urinate pretty much disappears the minute a bedpan appears, whether you are in labour or not. If you can't pee at all, you will be catheterised (and this will happen to all women having epidurals) which is not as unpleasant as it sounds and preferable to having a raging urinary infection afterwards.

13

Induction

*'I had piles, heartburn, I looked like a Michelin man and I
was a week overdue. When the man said, "We'd like to
induce you," I could have kissed him.'*

I must be honest and say that when I was planning this book,
induction of labour wasn't high on my list of priority chapters.
But that was before the survey results came in. Induction
didn't appear in the 'worries' section, but it appeared time and
time again in the 'I wish I'd known' part of the survey.

*'Nobody told me that the pain of inducement would be
worse than the labour itself.'*

Induction of labour is an obstetric procedure which is
designed to pre-empt the natural process of labour by initiating
its onset artificially before it occurs spontaneously. The
decision to induce labour is usually taken to serve some
interest, most usually that of the baby, less often that of the
mother and sometimes that of the obstetrician and medical
service. Few issues have generated as much controversy as this
one, particularly in the days when the ability to induce labour
seemed to outstrip sound clinical judgement. So let's first look
at some of the reasons why labour might be induced.

It is rare these days for labour induction to have to be
considered with regard to the mother's health. In years past, if

women had a chronic medical condition, such as heart or kidney disease, they were advised not to have children and, if they got pregnant, to have a termination. The worry was always that the additional stress of pregnancy might cause a dangerous deterioration in their condition. The new methods of inducing labour allow obstetricians to interrupt a pregnancy if and when it threatens the mother's life, and not before – and hopefully at a stage when the baby is sufficiently advanced to have a good chance of healthy survival.

Intervention can only ever be appropriate when its risks are judged to be fewer than those which might result if no intervention is made. There are certainly pregnancy complications which carry clearcut risks for the baby – rhesus disease, diabetes and severe pre-eclampsia being the most obvious examples. Yet even in these situations the decision when to deliver the baby is not easy. It's a constant balance of risks: yes, the rhesus baby may be becoming more and more anaemic, but deliver the baby too soon and it may die, not of anaemia, but from complications associated with prematurity.

One fairly common reason for induction is that the baby is overdue, but the evidence for induction here is even less clearcut. Some obstetricians are fairly relaxed about babies being overdue, regarding it as a variation of normal and following a policy of 'expectant management'. Others are much keener to end pregnancy at 'term', i.e. at 40 weeks, especially for pregnancies in older women. And there is no doubt that some doctors employ emotional blackmail, suggesting that a woman's failure to agree to induction will put her baby at risk. Women themselves are evenly divided about induction on these grounds; at 42 weeks, an equal proportion will accept and refuse induction. Only 4 per cent of babies are born on the due delivery date. Whilst some women are happy to wait, others find the days after that magic date are quite interminable. Your friends won't help either, saying things like, 'Are you still here?'

Being past your delivery date doesn't win prizes for comfort for sure, but what is the evidence for it being harmful to the baby? The justification for induction is that in the past there was a clear increase in baby deaths associated with being born past term. However, these figures were skewed by the inclusion of babies with particular types of lethal handicap, most notably anencephaly, which are associated with a prolonged pregnancy. These conditions were not detected antenatally as they would be today. There is no scientific justification for a policy of delivering all babies electively after 280 days (40 weeks) in order to prevent post-term pregnancy altogether. But the evidence thereafter, one way or another, is either lacking altogether or very scanty. If you are happy to sit it out, however, you might feel more reassured if you had monitoring every couple of days or so.

There are one or two myths about induction that are worth scotching. One is that women are more likely to have caesareans; this simply isn't borne out by the figures. Also, it is always said that induced labour is likely to be more painful and that there is therefore a higher rate of epidural use. Whilst the former statement may have some truth, the latter does not, which is surprising given that epidurals are more likely to be available during working hours, when inductions are most likely to be carried out.

Over the years, many women have given me their suggestions as to how to get labour started naturally. The Parry personal recipe is a stiff gin and tonic, followed by a blinding curry, and if you can manage it, bonk for Britain afterwards. The only element here with any science behind it is the bonking. Semen contains prostaglandins (hromone-like substances). Prostaglandins, it appears, are the pump primers as far as getting the womb into contraction mode is concerned. They also play a central role in 'ripening' of the cervix. Incidentally, oxytocin is also released naturally when you twiddle your nipples in late pregnancy (as you do) and someone undertook a trial showing that women who spent an average of three hours a day either twiddling their nipples or (and this is the bit I prefer) having them twiddled for them, went into labour significantly earlier than women who didn't nipple-twiddle. I suppose it occupies the day.

You may hear all sorts of other things suggested such as taking purgatives like castor oil. The thought here is that the unpleasant attack of diarrhoea that may follow might precipitate labour. On the other hand, you might still have an unshiftable bulge and be constantly running up and down stairs to the loo. In all seriousness, I wouldn't recommend this sort of approach; nasty diarrhoea can leave you feeling weak and debilitated and that's the last way you want to feel when you go into labour.

'The worst thing about my second pregnancy was thinking that it might be as much overdue as the first one was. The first one was 11 days overdue, and the second one 15 days. I resorted to cycling in the end.'

If you think about it, your womb and cervix have to reverse their roles completely during labour. The womb has to go from being a muscular holding bag that does not contract, to being a bag that contracts so much that the contents are expelled. And the cervix has to go from being a rigid plug, to being soft and pliant. Although this process may seem to be a sudden one, in reality it is the culmination of a gradual process evolving over a period of weeks. During this period of pre-labour, the womb practises contractions and the cervix 'ripens'. This curious obstetric expression means that the cervix softens itself so that, when the moment arrives, it will be able to dilate rapidly.

There are only three broad approaches to induction of labour: sweeping of the membranes (also called stripping), amniotomy (breaking the membranes) and the use of drugs such as prostaglandins or oxytocin.

You could pump in oxytocin (the hormone used to speed up labour) by the truckload early in pregnancy and it would have no effect. But the womb can be made responsive to oxytocin if prostaglandins (which are hormone-like sub-stances) are administered first. In some ways all labour induction is really labour acceleration because all it is doing is bringing forward an inevitable prospect. The method of induction that is used is dependent on where you are on the continuum − pregnancy, pre-labour, latent labour (i.e. when you've started and then stopped again), active labour, delivery − and the closer you are to labour proper, the easier it is going to be to induce labour.

> 'The midwife said it wasn't going to hurt. I just went through the roof. She then told me I was being a silly girl.'

'Sweeping' involves inserting a finger through the cervix and sweeping it around between the membranes and the womb. Some people say it can be painful. It can be quite excruciating. Often sweeping is enough to set you off in labour and it's usually done in the hope that pessaries and the like can be avoided in the very late stages of pregnancy.

If you are still some weeks away from your delivery date and need to be induced, or even if you are at term but just have a baby that won't budge, techniques such as this are no good. Even if you went into labour, the cervix wouldn't be ready to dilate. Thus, before the pharmaceutical big guns can be brought in, the cervix needs to be 'ripened' by using prostaglandins. These substances are not circulating hormones, like oestrogen, but are produced very close to the organ that they act upon. Because of the speed with which circulating prostaglandins are rendered inactive, doses given by mouth have, of necessity, to be very large and may provoke troublesome side effects. One way to overcome this, however, is to give smaller doses of prostaglandin very frequently – say one tablet every hour. But most prostaglandins are administered as vaginal pessaries or gels. The most familiar brand names you will hear are Prostin, Cervagem or Prepidil (a gel).

> *'I got the giggles when they broke my waters. There was so much fluid, the consultant said he could have floated the Britannia on it. Lucky he was wearing wellingtons.'*

Once your cervix has begun to dilate, your membranes may be broken. This is called by various names – artificial rupture of the membranes (ARM) or amniotomy, in which a special hook is used. It is quite likely that this is all you will need to put you into strong labour. There is usually a noticeable change of gear once the waters have broken, partly because the baby is now pressing directly on the cervix instead of having a cushion of fluid to press on, and labour may become a lot more intense and painful for some women at this stage. Actually even if women are in established early labour, their waters will probably be broken. There are no sense endings in the amniotic sac and therefore amniotomy is painless.

> *'I was induced and had the works, Syntocinon, epidural, everything. My husband and I sat and played Monopoly*

and occasionally one of us would look at the trace, and say "Look, here's another contraction." It was the only way I knew I was having them! It was bliss compared to my first "natural labour". But seeing how close those lines were together, I don't think I could have coped without the epidural.'

The final weapon in the induction armoury is the hormone oxytocin. In the same way that amniotomy wouldn't be any good prior to use of prostaglandins, oxytocin won't work before the membranes are broken. It would seem that when the membranes break, the womb suddenly becomes receptive to oxytocin. Oxytocin is more likely to be used when your waters have gone, but you haven't yet gone into labour. It is also used extensively to augment labour if it has slowed down. It is usually administered as an intravenous infusion controlled by a mechanical infusion pump. Synthetic oxytocin is dispensed under its brand name, Syntocinon. The dosage is started at a fairly low rate and then built up gradually. When oxytocin is used, the baby will be monitored continuously using a fetal scalp electrode, because the strength of the artificial contractions may affect it.

There is no doubt that an oxytocin-speeded labour is likely to be more intense and 80 per cent of women will find it more painful. It will also be restricted in that, because you will be attached to the drip, you will not be able to move around in the same way as if you were unattached. If you are having an oxytocin drip to speed up a slow labour, you might like to try some other methods first – like walking around, or having something to drink and eat (providing it is light), as this may do the trick. You might think that an oxytocin-augmented labour is shorter, but one study has shown that a control group in which women were mobile in labour had shorter labour times than the drug-augmented group. It is also the case that about half of women judged to have slow labours or poor progress in cervical dilatation will progress equally well whether or not oxytocic drugs are given. But remember, half of them needed the oxytocic drugs.

I do not personally believe that induction for social reasons (to fit in with the consultant's golf) is practised on a wide scale in NHS hospitals in Britain now. It is rife in private hospitals, but women who use private maternity services seem to regard this as part of the deal. If you pay your money and have a fancy obstetrician, you don't want a lesser mortal delivering your baby just because you inconveniently go into labour when God is on holiday. After all, what have you paid good money for? A more likely type of social induction in the NHS is where a woman likely to have a particularly complicated birth (e.g. multiple delivery) is induced in order to ensure that a full complement of staff is available, but I think this is acceptable.

You might read all of this and think that induction is something very nasty that you would rather avoid if you can. Certainly many survey respondents said that they were worried about induction. Of course spontaneous labour is to be preferred, but sometimes things just don't work out this way. You may feel that your body has let you down or that things would have been a great deal better had you had a normal labour, and feel disappointed and sad about it. But what would have happened had you not had an induced labour? It might not have been half so rosy as you imagine.

Let me put the other side of the coin to you. Pay a visit to the museum of the Royal College of Obstetricians and you will see all sorts of deeply unpleasant mechanical devices used to force open the cervix, to deliver babies prior to spontaneous labour, in eras when caesarean section was still very dangerous. The result was predictable. The baby died, and if the mother lived she would have a cervix which would never again stand the strain of full term pregnancy. Induction as we know it now is an advance which has saved thousands and thousands of lives. My feeling is that if you are offered an induction for what seem to be good reasons, accept it and don't fret over it. Be positive about its benefits, such as seeing light at the end of a long pregnancy. Use the time advantage that induction gives you to be prepared in terms of pain relief, e.g. epidural, and remember above all that whilst birth might be a life experience, it is a transient one compared to the lifetime you will experience with your child.

14

Having a Caesarean Section

At least 1 in 10 women will deliver her baby by caesarean section, and in some hospitals the caesarean section rate may be as high as 1 in 5 deliveries. Women ought to be aware of the possibility of their pregnancy ending in a caesarean section. Certainly, 20 per cent of respondents to our survey reported themselves as being 'very worried' that this might happen to them. And, in line with national statistics, 11 per cent of those who were very worried did indeed have a section. But what was most interesting of all was that, despite your fears, despite knowing how common section is, 14 per cent of all our respondents – which probably represents nearly all those who had caesareans – felt completely unprepared for their delivery.

Of course some people know almost from the outset that they will be having an elective caesarean i.e. one that is arranged in advance of them going into labour. In about 6 per cent of deliveries, there is an absolute necessity for a caesarean section; there simply isn't an alternative. Some, like a small pelvis as revealed by a previous birth, are known in advance. Others, like placenta praevia, are not known until later in pregnancy. However, there are many pregnancy/birth problems for which a caesarean is not mandatory, simply a matter of medical opinion, with different hospitals and doctors adopting different practices according to their views and training. For instance, babies usually turn head down fairly late in pregnancy. When women go into labour too soon, the baby is very often in a breech position (bottom down). Whilst some obstetricians would always undertake a caesarean for a premature breech, others would not. There isn't a right or wrong here because there is no clearcut scientific evidence to justify one approach over the other. There are just two schools of thought.

Here then, are some of the indications for caesareans. I have made clear where a section might be a matter of opinion, and where it is essential.

Placenta Praevia and Other Placental and Cord Problems

If the placenta is blocking the baby's exit from the womb, a condition called placenta praevia, an elective caesarean is essential. A low lying placenta is often diagnosed in early pregnancy, whilst true placenta praevia is uncommon. Read Chapter 7 on placenta praevia for further details. If the baby is still alive after a placental abruption (when the placenta separates partially or totally from the womb wall) a section is indicated. If your waters have broken, and if the baby's head isn't engaged properly, the cord may fall out of the womb, and even out of the vagina, ahead of the baby. Without emergency sections in both these cases, the baby will die because its blood supply is being obstructed.

Problems with the Mother's Health

The course of pre-eclampsia, the pregnancy disease most often characterised by high blood pressure, protein in the urine and oedema, is very unpredictable. The only 'cure' is to deliver the baby. As you will read in Chapter 11, women very often feel perfectly well when they have pre-eclampsia, and you may feel that your carers are making a ridiculous fuss. A caesarean may be suggested and you may resist it, feeling that it can't possibly be necessary for someone as healthy as you. If pre-eclampsia gets out of hand – and the fact that you already have high blood pressure, etc., is an indication that the condition is unstable – there is a real risk that you may lose your baby, and your life may also be on the line. Speed is of the essence, hence the emergency caesarean. Some other maternal conditions, such as heart disease, may also make elective caesarean a possibility.

Not Enough Room for the Baby

I have already compared the pelvis to a bucket without a bottom. Obviously if the baby's head (its widest part) is bigger than the hole at the bottom of the bucket, it cannot get out. 'Obstructed labours' used to be far more common than they are today, partly because diseases which affect the shape and size of the pelvis, such as rickets, were rife. The medical term for 'not enough room' is cephalo-pelvic disproportion. Women often say that they feel that doctors should have known there was a problem with cephalo-pelvic disproportion before they went into labour. In truth, it is notoriously difficult to assess. Even with ultrasound assessment of the baby's weight and head measurements, and knowledge of the mother's pelvis (either through clinical examination or X-ray), it is not always possible to predict the outcome. Thus, unless a woman's pelvis is clearly shown to be too small, the balance of evidence is in favour of encouraging a woman to deliver vaginally. In any case, the baby's head is the best assessor of the size of its mother's pelvis.

Just because you are little and your husband is big or tall, does not necessarily mean that you will have a baby which is too big. The baby's size is limited by your dimensions, for a start. There used to be much tut-tutting over women who had a small shoe-size relative to their height, and shoe-size therefore used to be a routine measurement at antenatal booking. No longer. Whilst it is true that short women, who may also have small feet, statistically have more caesarean sections, there is such a huge overlap in obstetric outcome between women with small and large dimensions that foot size is no more relevant than asking which supermarket you do your weekly shop at. Occasionally cephalo-pelvic disproportion can arise in a woman who has had one or more babies without problem before, either because this baby is much bigger, or because of some other difficulty.

One thing which may alert your carers in advance to possible disproportion is late engagement of the head. Normally, the baby's head descends down into the bucket, that is the pelvis, until the head is tucked snugly at the bottom of the bucket ready for delivery. In first pregnancies the head may engage from about 30 weeks onwards and is usually fully engaged two to three weeks before delivery. In subsequent pregnancies, the head may not engage fully until just before labour. There is always a suspicion that if a baby's head hasn't engaged it is because it can't engage because the pelvis is too narrow. There is an easy way to check this. You will be asked to lie on your back. In this position your carer will be able to feel your baby's head resting at the brim of the pelvis. You will then be asked to prop yourself up on your elbows. In this position the baby's head should, if there is no problem, slip into the pelvis.

There are some other situations where a caesarean is necessary because of the way in which the baby is lying in the womb. A transverse lie – where the baby is lying across the womb, instead of head down – is one of these. Many obstetricians, as indicated previously, would regard a breech position (bottom down instead of head down) as a reason for a section. However, there is controversy about this. In the past, obstetricians tried to turn babies – a process called external version – by manipulating a woman's pregnant abdomen before 36 weeks. This practice fell into disfavour, partly because the baby so often turned back itself. However, external version is now being revived, and is undertaken after relaxing the womb with drugs at about 37 weeks or more (i.e. at term). This type of external version signficantly reduces the incidence of breech presentation and can reduce the rate of caesarean section by half. You should be aware that this practice is regarded as an invasive procedure, since there is risk for the baby (there will be a placental abruption – see pages 128–32 – in 1 in 100 women having external version) and you should discuss it fully with your carers.

There are said to be several non-invasive ways of turning uncooperative babies. Some people advocate the mother adopting a knee-chest position (kneeling, but with the head and shoulders flat on the floor) on a daily basis, which is supposed to allow the baby space to turn. The single proper trial of this approach reported only a 10 per cent reversal rate, which wasn't statistically significant (it could have been due to chance alone). Another ploy is to dive repeatedly to the bottom of the deep end of a swimming pool, allowing gravity to come to your aid (the theory is that the baby's head – its heaviest part – will naturally turn in this situation). Talking about this on a TV show one day, I said that, although there were no guarantees it would work, women could try it if they wanted. 'And of course,' I added, 'there's no risk.' Quick as a flash, the presenter came back, 'But there's a hell of a problem if you can't swim.' He was right; not a good one to try if you can't swim.

What you need to remember is that 25 per cent of babies are breech before 30 weeks, but that only 3 per cent of babies are breech at full term. If you are 36 weeks with a breech baby, read about caesareans but don't assume that it will necessarily end this way.

Problems with the Baby

A constant problem for obstetricians is deciding whether babies in the womb are little and healthy or little and sick. The difference is crucial because the little, sick babies may have used up all their reserves of energy and may not survive the rigours of a vaginal delivery. These are babies that need to be delivered by caesarean. Babies that seem not to be moving as much as they were, or perhaps don't seem to be moving at all, also need to be carefully monitored using electronic fetal monitoring and also Doppler ultrasound scanning. This latter technique uses the same principles as ultrasound scanning, but instead of a picture, you get a pattern on a screen. The pattern is related to bloodflow in the different blood vessels supplying the placenta and baby. Babies are capable, as a last ditch effort when they are in desperate trouble, of reversing the flow in the blood vessels in their necks, in an effort to divert blood preferentially to the brain. A baby seen doing this on Doppler scan needs to be rescued fast.

About 1 in 100 babies will show signs of acute distress during labour. A larger number will show some signs of fetal distress – such as abnormalities in the heart rate, or passing meconium (the contents of the bowel) but this does not necessarily mean that a caesarean is indicated. Sometimes the solution is simple. For instance, the woman's position may mean that the womb is pressing on the blood return to her heart, which is in turn giving the baby problems. Shifting position slightly may sort this out.

Nobody wants to waste time if the baby is in trouble, but electronic monitoring can cause false alarms, partly because the traces are sometimes quite difficult to interpret. Fetal blood sampling is a better way of checking how much oxygen is available to the baby, but not all hospitals have the facility to do this.

Long, Difficult Labours

The medical name for a long and difficult labour is dystocia. There is considerable variation in what is termed long. A twelve-hour labour seemed pretty monumental to me, but 'long' labours can be anything up to thirty-six hours. If you talk to women of your mother's generation, they will often speak of labours lasting several days. There are a variety of reasons why labour can be slow. The womb may not be contracting efficiently. The cervix may not dilate properly. The baby may not be in the right position. There may be cephalo-pelvic disproportion. Slow labour in itself isn't necessarily a cause for concern, provided that both mother and baby are well. About half the women judged to have slow labour or poor cervical dilatation will progress equally well whether or not drugs such as oxytocin, which strengthen the contractions, are administered. Rupturing the membranes may be sufficient to speed things up. But for those women where labour comes to a halt, for those where labour just isn't getting anywhere, and for those where exhaustion and distress have set in, caesarean section may be the only option.

For many women, a long exhausting labour followed by a caesarean is the worst of all worlds. There is a suspicion that some sections in this category could be avoided and that some are undertaken because they are the quick easy option when mothers could, if they were left longer or the labour was better managed, deliver vaginally. This might be true in general. On the other hand, in your own case, it might not. And anyone who has been at the receiving end of a long difficult labour will tell you that the only thing they wanted after twenty-nine hours in labour was for it to end *right now*. Afterwards, the initial feeling of relief at it all being over may recede, and you may feel miserable and guilty, thinking that if only you'd done something different or been a bit less of a wimp you could have done it on your own. Theory might say you could. Real life is different. Don't torture yourself.

Previous Surgery

If you have had surgery for a prolapse, for a fistula, or any type of surgery aimed at correcting incontinence, elective caesarean section will be suggested, as vaginal delivery may make further surgery necessary.

Herpes

It is not uncommon for women to suffer from genital herpes during pregnancy, either a recurrent attack or for the first time. In America, the policy is that women with a history of genital herpes should be screened throughout the latter part of pregnancy and delivered by caesarean either if there is a positive culture or if genital lesions are present within a week of delivery. Some American physicians recommend an elective section for all women with a history of herpes. In Britain, where genital herpes is far less prevalent (a third of pregnant US women have antibodies to the herpes virus, compared to an average of 10 per cent in British women), policy varies but many hospitals would only suggest a caesarean if there were genital lesions at the time of delivery.

If a baby is infected by the herpes virus and it spreads throughout its body, about 80 per cent of such babies would die without treatment and the rest have severe, long-term damage to many organs, particularly the eyes and brain. Antiviral therapy is available, but even so, 20 per cent still die.

About 1 in 40,000 live births in the UK will have neonatal herpes, so this is a rare disease. On average only sixteen cases are reported each year. Neonatal herpes might be rare but, as I have indicated, genital herpes is not. About 12,000 cases are reported each year through specialist clinics, and clearly a great many more cases remain unreported. A caesarean section might be mentioned if you have herpes, so you need to know the odds. For a start, less than 30 per cent of the mothers of the 71 babies recorded as having neonatal herpes between July 1986 and December 1991 had a past history of genital herpes, or any evidence of a recurrent or primary infection. At one centre in California, 34 infants exposed to herpes during delivery were identified. Half their mothers had active lesions, yet none of the babies developed neonatal herpes. American data now suggest that even when there are lesions, provided they are recurrent, there is little risk to the baby because of the protective effect of neutralising antibody. The advice of the Public Health Laboratory Service is that caesarean section is only necessary when primary infection is present at delivery, and even then only if the membranes have been ruptured for less than four hours.

One final, nothing to do with caesareans, note about herpes. If either you or your partner have an active herpes infection, for instance a cold sore, you should be absolutely scrupulous about not touching or cuddling newborn babies other than your own. Your baby has antibodies to herpes acquired through you; the baby you are touching may not have this advantage and could be infected by you. This route of infection is probably much more likely than infection through delivery.

Premature or Multiple Pregnancies

For babies likely to weigh less than 1500 g (3 lbs 6 oz) at birth, caesarean section seems to offer some advantages in terms of survival rate, whereas the survival rate for babies weighing more than this is not affected by their mode of delivery. Of course this assumes that the baby's weight can be accurately determined antenatally, which is not always the case. In practice, this would occur in pregnancies complicated by antepartum haemorrhage or pre-eclampsia. Higher order births, such as triplets and quads are usually delivered by caesarean.

Repeat Caesareans

There used to be an edict: 'once a caesarean always a caesarean'. This pronouncement was made at a time when the usual incision was a vertical one (running up and down rather than across the abdomen). The concern was that subsequent labour might rupture the scar and it was assumed that repeat caesareans would be safer. In fact, the chance of a woman dying from problems associated with caesarean section such as anaesthetic reactions or pulmonary embolism is very small (40 per 100,000 births overall), but it is still considerably higher than with vaginal delivery (10 per 100,000 births overall), which is therefore always to be preferred if possible. Assuming that repeat elective caesareans are safer does not bear up to scrutiny. True, the death rate drops (to 18 per 100,000 births), but the comparable figure for straightforward normal vaginal deliveries is just 5 per 100,000.

Of course, some reasons for caesareans, such as placenta praevia or placental abruption, have only a small risk of occurring in a subsequent pregnancy. The greatest likelihood of a successful vaginal delivery following a caesarean is seen when the first section was undertaken because of breech presentation. Vaginal delivery rates are lowest when the initial indication was failure to progress in labour or disproportion. However, even when the reason for the first section was disproportion, a difficult labour or failure to progress, vaginal delivery occurred in over 50 per cent of the time, with over 75 per cent being successful in the largest series of cases reported. Women who have had a previous vaginal delivery, in addition to one or more sections, have the highest success rate of subsequent vaginal delivery of all. But in truth, there's not that much between these figures and the likelihood of vaginal delivery is not significantly altered either by the indication for the first section nor by a history of more than one section.

What of the worry about rupturing the uterus? It is a concern if the previous section used a classical or low vertical incision, and in most cases this is a contra-indication to a trial of labour (allowing a woman to proceed with labour, to see whether she can deliver vaginally, rather than forestalling labour with a caesarean). But the probability of a woman requiring an emergency caesarean in her next delivery for other acute conditions (such as prolapsed cord, haemorrhage, fetal distress, etc.) is actually, to put it in perspective, 2.7 per cent or 30 times as high as the risk of a uterine rupture during a trial of labour. In any case, even if a lower segment scar did rupture, a hospital equipped to deal with the usual run of obstetric dramas should be able to cope. I think it is well worth trying labour.

Having a Caesarean

About 60 per cent of women have a general anaesthetic, with 40 per cent opting to be awake, choosing an epidural or a spinal block. For women having an emergency section there may be no option but to proceed to a general anaesthetic. For most women having elective sections there is a choice. In many ways, an epidural is to be preferred because a general anaesthetic tends to make people feel rather drowsy and disorientated for a day or two. It also means that your partner and you can share the experience (partners are often excluded when a general anaesthetic is used). The epidural tube can also be left in place and can be used for very effective pain relief post-operatively. The best thing is that you will be awake to hear your baby's first cry, and to welcome him into the world. However, you may be completely squeamish about being awake whilst having major surgery, and if this is the case don't feel pressurised into having an epidural.

Some women having an emergency section will already have an epidural in place and this can simply be topped up with a larger dose of anaesthetic to give total pain relief. If you need an emergency section and have a general anaesthetic, you will be given an antacid to drink, which will minimise the risk of your stomach contents reaching your lungs and causing

problems. In addition, drugs may be given to neutralise the
stomach contents. The anaesthetic will go into your arm via a
small tube and takes about thirty seconds to work. The
anaesthetist may press on your neck during this time – yet
another move to prevent acid stomach contents reaching your
lungs.

You will discover that suddenly the room is full of people
– an anaesthetist, an obstetrician, plus a more junior member
of the obstetric team, a paediatrician (to check the condition of
the baby after birth), and an assortment of midwives and
nurses. If there is time, your pubic hair will have been shaved.
For elective sections, an enema may have been given. Unless
there is a pressing medical reason to do otherwise, virtually all
incisions are horizontal, just below the line of the pubic hair.
Your bladder will be emptied with a catheter and you may
find that this is left in place for a bit after the caesarean in some
hospitals. A screen will be erected just over your chest. This is
not so that you can't see what is going on. It is actually to
protect you from the diathermy equipment – special heat-
sealing equipment which will be used to close off small blood
vessels and thus control bleeding. Usually every effort is made
to explain what is going on to both you and your partner.

The general anaesthetic given is quite light and women
may be aware of lights and voices, but feel no pain. For those
having an epidural, there are odd sensations – stretching and
tickling – but no pain.

The abdomen is swabbed with coloured antiseptic before a
horizontal incision about five inches long is made at the top of
the hairline. The bladder, which lies on top of the womb, is
pushed to one side. A second incision in the wall of the womb
is then made and both incisions are cauterised to prevent blood
loss. Amniotic fluid is pumped out before the baby is
delivered. Some women may be aware of warm fluid on their

legs as the second incision is made (I just say this because should you be one of those that feels fluid you may otherwise think it must be blood, and that you are bleeding to death). The baby's head will be lifted through the incision by the obstetrician, either using one hand or using forceps, whilst an assistant presses down on the top of the abdomen to help ease the baby's body out. If the baby is lying the other way around, the legs are lifted out first and forceps used to cradle the head during delivery. The umbilical cord is then clamped. It will take about five minutes to do all of this.

Babies are designed to be born via the vagina. For instance, the amniotic fluid contained in their lungs is cleared as the baby passes down the birth canal and their circulation is also stimulated. Thus, babies born by section may need resuscitation and some extra care and attention after delivery. Their breathing may not start for a minute or two but this is not dangerous. Not all babies cry immediately at birth, so the fact that your baby may be quiet is nothing to worry about. The plus of caesarean section as far as babies are concerned is that they end up looking far less squashed.

If you have had an epidural you will be given the baby to hold. If you are having a general your partner may be given your baby at this point if he is close by. The placenta is then removed and an injection of Syntometrine given to minimise the risk of heavy bleeding from the womb. If you have had an elective caesarean (i.e. haven't gone into labour), the cervix may be dilated to allow blood to drain into the vagina. After the baby has been delivered, the amount of anaesthetic (general and epidural) is increased and the task of sewing you up begins. This takes far longer than delivering the baby – about forty minutes.

The incision in the womb is stitched up with dissolving stitches (sutures). The bladder is put back in the right place and then the skin wound is closed either by little curved staples or by a fancy bit of surgeon's embroidery, a sort of hidden running stitch kept in place by beads at either end of the wound. A drain may be placed in the incision to remove liquid and the wound then covered with either gauze or sticky plaster. (Incidentally, when you first book always declare an allergy to zinc oxide plasters, however slight, as otherwise, like me, you may come home with dramatic weals where you've had standard-issue hospital plasters stuck in unexpected places.)

If you have had a general, you will be taken to a recovery room. When awake you will be shown your baby, although you may not remember this as you may go straight back to sleep again, finding yourself in the ward the next time you wake up. You may feel a bit sick from the anaesthetic but there are drugs which will help you with this. You may be attached to a drip. This will replace fluid, as you won't be able to drink right away (otherwise you'll be sick). You may find that you have a catheter which is attached to a bottle or bag under the bed. All these tubes may be a bit alarming if you are not prepared for them, but they will soon go – the fluid drip will disappear after 12–24 hours. Painkillers may also be given by a drip, or by injection into your buttock or thigh. In general, oral painkillers will not be used for a day or so because your digestive system 'shuts down' after an operation, especially an abdominal one, and the drugs will not be absorbed properly.

This is not a time for heroics. You've had major surgery. You wouldn't expect a woman who had had a hysterectomy to cope without pain relief; you've had a very similar bit of surgery – so if you are in pain tell someone and they'll arrange appropriate pain relief.

You will probably find that you suffer from wind after a section and your stomach may swell because of the air trapped in the abdomen during the operation. This will pass, literally, when you open your bowels. You may also have heartburn. Some hospitals have cocktails, once you can drink, that contain peppermint water (a sovereign remedy for wind) together with soluble painkillers. These painkillers are only transferred to breast milk in minute quantities, so are safe for breastfeeding mothers to use. Please don't try to cope without pain relief in the belief that it is better for your baby.

Women who have had an epidural may find that the epidural tube is left in place for twenty-four hours and this provides very effective pain relief. Some women use the TENS machine they have hired for labour for relief.

You will be given a short course of antibiotics which, given prophylactically in this way, have been shown to reduce post-partum infection dramatically amongst women who have had sections. Again, the antibiotics that are used only get through to breastmilk in minute quantities, so don't worry.

You'll be allowed to drink the day following the operation and usually to eat the day after that. It is very important, however rotten you feel and no matter how sadistic you think the nurses are, that you try to get up and about as soon as possible. This will ensure that your circulation gets moving, it will get your digestion going again and help relieve any wind pains. The quicker you are up and about, the quicker you will get better.

You should have the earliest possible access to a physiotherapist who will show you how to guard your wound and become mobile. She will make you cough, showing you first how to support your scar when you do so, to help clear your chest. This is particularly important if you have had a general anaesthetic. You will find that it takes a very long time even to get to the loo at first, and that you may need someone with you to make sure you are all right. Try to stand as upright as you can before you start to walk. Walking all hunched up may seem like a good idea, but actually it doesn't help as gravity will be pulling your internal organs against your scar. You may feel as if everything is about to drop out, but it won't. Use your breathing and relaxation techniques to stop yourself tensing up as this will increase your pain.

Getting in and out of bed won't be easy the first few times. The best way to do it is to roll onto your side with your knees bent, then raise yourself on your elbow and swing your legs over the side of the bed, pushing yourself into a sitting position with your arms. To get back into bed, simply reverse the procedure: sit on the edge of the bed, lower yourself sideways using your arms and swing your legs up as you do this, then roll onto your back.

You badly need to sleep and you should take every opportunity to do so. The staff will probably offer to change and settle your baby and bring him to you only when he needs feeding. If you would prefer to keep your baby beside you, don't try to get him out of the cot yourself at first – ask for help.

After a couple of days or so, you may be offered a shower or bath. The shower may be preferable if you find bending over very painful. The wound heals best if kept as dry as possible, so a good soak is out. Scrupulous hygiene is essential and if you are having a bath, ask someone to clean it for you first. If you are one of those unfortunate women who has stitches (from a trial by forceps) as well as a caesarean wound, read Chapter 17 on afterbirth care.

You will need to wear a sanitary towel, because you will still be losing blood (the technical name is lochia) from inside the womb, as you would have had you had a normal delivery. However, you will need to experiment with knickers which do not chafe your wound. Men's paper knickers are good. If you find yourself in hospital over a holiday weekend, with all the shops shut, and you having had an emergency section, your partner's knickers are more likely to fulfil the brief (if you'll excuse the pun) than any you have. If your lochia becomes at all smelly or offensive, you should tell someone.

Breast feeding is more difficult than after normal deliveries, not because breast feeding itself is a problem, but because you are trying to cope with the after-effects of major surgery as well. The NCT do a range of very good leaflets on breast feeding, including some that are designed specifically for women who have had sections. Finding a position that is comfortable is all important. Underarm positions (where the baby is lying on a pillow) may be best. It is especially important for someone to check that the baby is latched on properly, because the pain that is caused when a baby isn't feeding properly, and that of sore nipples, may not be apparent because of the pain relief you are having.

You may find that it takes longer for your breast milk to come in – sometimes as long as five or six days. This may be partly because you have been denied food and drink for two or three days, and partly because you have a drowsy baby who is sucking less strongly than an alert baby. You may also be reluctant to put the baby to the breast as frequently as other mothers because of the discomfort it causes your scar – hence the importance of finding a comfortable position. Your baby will not suffer because of the delay in your milk coming in, and is having colostrum, which is richer than milk, in the meantime. You should not be tempted to let your baby have supplementary feeds because it will only delay your milk further. In any case it's highly likely that you are doing just fine on your own.

There is a breast feeding lobby that suggests that unless babies are put to the breast directly after birth breast feeding is unlikely to establish itself properly. Women who have had a section under general anaesthetic may feel in consequence that their breast feeding is unlikely to be successful. Actually, there are millions of women worldwide who, for religious reasons, do not start breast feeding until the milk proper comes in. They are perfectly good breastfeeders.

After five days your stitches will be removed and you will be allowed to go home. All those things which are outlined in Chapter 17 on 'afterwards' apply, but with knobs on. You have had major surgery and need all the rest and help you can get. A stream of visitors is out – it's just too exhausting. You will also need to arrange help at home, especially if you have other children. Perhaps your mother could stay for a few days. You will not be able to lift for at least six weeks – which means, for instance, not attempting to get your hulk of a three-year-old out of the bath, nor attempting to lift the shopping out of the car. It is also advised that you should not drive for six weeks in case you have to brake suddenly and put excessive strain on your scar. You may however find that not being able to drive puts an excessive strain on you if you have to use the bus instead, so compromise. Return to driving gradually, and get other people to ferry you about or do the school run whenever possible. You certainly shouldn't drive at all for 2–3 weeks.

If you are on your own, for whatever reason, tell your community midwife who may be able to get you some help. Your first consideration should be the baby; everything else can either wait, or someone can do it for you.

You will find that your scar will gradually fade, although it may go through a period of being very itchy. Vitamin E cream or wheatgerm oil should help. It is usual for there to be a little numb patch around the scar for a while. Some people find that this is permanent. You will have a six week postnatal check in the same way as other mothers, but if you want to have a coil fitted you will have to wait until three months after the birth.

Coping

Having a baby is a pretty dramatic event: there are huge swings in hormones to cope with, your emotions threaten to overwhelm you, there's this tiny baby to care for, and what's more you are completely exhausted. For the woman who has had a caesarean, you have to add to this heady brew the effects of major abdominal surgery with its attendant discomfort and possible infection. Small wonder that women having caesareans are more likely to suffer from postnatal depression than those who have delivered vaginally. It doesn't help either that all your friends seem to have got back to normal in no time, whilst here you are, still unable to lift heavy loads, still not driving and possibly still hurting as well. It doesn't seem fair.

The emotional aftermath of a caesarean is probably as significant as the physical one. You may have had a very long and difficult labour, followed by a dramatic caesarean, and have been totally drained of emotion, with nothing left for the baby. About 40 per cent of mothers find that the overwhelming feelings of love they expected to feel took several days to develop. So don't expect it all at once – it's perfectly normal for it to take time to get to know your baby. In addition, if your section was an emergency, you may feel cheated in some way, that you aren't a 'proper' mother because you haven't given birth, and that your body let you down. Again, such feelings of disappointment and even of failure are common and it may help you to talk them over with other women who have had caesareans. Your partner may understand but, standing on the other side of the fence as it were, having perhaps seen you at your wits' end, and having been more aware than perhaps you were of the danger that the baby faced, he may not appreciate why you feel as you do. If you are still feeling angry and depressed about your birth, talk to your consultant. Ask him to tell you how it was and explain why the caesarean was necessary. Asking all the questions you want and understanding why you had to have a section may make you feel better about it.

The thing to remember is that the way you gave birth is not a reflection on your abilities as a mother. You became a mother when the baby was born and your relationship grows from that day on, and keeps on growing. You may feel bad about the section – but it matters not a jot to your baby.

Finally, a word about the origin of the word 'caesarean'. It is assumed that the word is derived from the manner of delivery, as reported by Pliny, of one Julius Caesar, conqueror of Britain. Pliny is the only one however who makes this assertion and he was notoriously hazy about things historical. In any case, the fact that Julius's mum was recorded as being alive and well at the time of his invasion of Britain in 55 BC almost certainly rules out a caesarean section, which in those days inevitably resulted in the death of the mother. The more likely explanation is that a Roman law, the lex caesarea, called for separate burial of mother and child in cases where women died in late pregnancy. The few babies that did survive were called caesones. So 'caesarean' is much more likely to have come from the name of the law, not from Julius Caesar who was born some 700 years after this law was first enacted. You may have ended up with a caesarean section, but cheer up; armed with this knowledge, you'll be brilliant at Trivial Pursuit.

15

Premature and Special Care Babies

'My baby had been five weeks in intensive care before my friends who were expecting at the same time as me started their first antenatal classes. I was totally unprepared.'

'You could have looked round the special care bit of the hospital, as well as the labour wards. I never did, because I thought I was unlikely to use it and I really regretted it when Emma was born at 28 weeks because I think I would have been less scared.'

Whilst the majority of women are prepared for a baby that might be overdue, very few, it would seem from our survey, are prepared for a baby that arrives too soon. But prematurity is far more common than many people realise, with 1 in 10 deliveries being of a premature baby. 'Prematurity' is defined as a baby that is born at or before 37 weeks. At 37 weeks, a baby may be little but does not usually require special care of the sort that people normally associate with prematurity. On the other hand, very low birthweight (VLBW) babies, weighing 1,500 g (3 lbs 6 oz) or less (the average British male baby weighs 3,333 g – 7 lbs 5 oz – at term), would normally be born before 32 weeks and require a great deal of specialist intensive care. However, also included in this VLBW category are babies who are at or near term but who, because of factors such as growth retardation in the womb, may be very small. The outlook for babies who are born at 28 weeks or more is usually very good indeed.

Having Contractions Pre-term

About half of all women admitted to hospital pre-term with regular contractions are not actually in labour. If the waters have not broken and there is little or no change to the cervix, neither the frequency and regularity of contractions, the level of discomfort, nor even the time that the contractions persist can be used readily to distinguish between women who are in false labour and those in true labour. So in this situation expect to be admitted to hospital for close observation and rest. You will be asked to lie on your left side, or propped up, since this increases bloodflow to the womb, rather than flat on your back. An intravenous drip may also be set up. It usually contains water, as the infusion of water may also improve bloodflow to the womb and quieten down the activity of the womb muscles. It is thought that it may also inhibit release of the hormone oxytocin which speeds labour. For 1 in 5 women, this combination of bed rest and hydration will result in the contractions stopping altogether.

Both your baby and your contracting womb will be monitored and your cervix will be checked at regular intervals. If the cervix is much more than 2 cm dilated, labour may be very difficult to stop because a well dilated cervix is a sign that labour is advanced. Rather like a runaway train, advanced labour is almost impossible to stop.

You will be asked to provide a mid-stream specimen of urine (MSU), and your vagina and cervix will be swabbed, in case infection is the reason why your womb has started contracting. It may seem self-evident, if you have a high temperature and an obvious infection, be it a urinary tract problem or chickenpox, that labour may be set off too soon but actually the problem is rather more subtle. Evidence has been accumulating for some time that labour can be precipitated by the activity of bacteria infecting the vagina. You might think that there is nothing to suggest that you have an infection of this sort – no discharge out of the ordinary – but sub-clinical infection (i.e. infection of which the mother is completely unaware) is now thought to play an important role in the causation of pre-term labour. There are currently a number of trials involving the routine use of antibiotics in pregnancy to see whether this reduces the number of babies born prematurely. If infection is the cause of the pre-term labour in your case, antibiotics may stop it more effectively than any other measure.

A sample of blood will be taken for a complete blood count, and in some British hospitals, and often routinely in the States, your cervix may also be swabbed with something that I can only describe as a vaginal dipstick, for the presence of fibronectin. This is one of a family of proteins found in placental tissue. It is thought that fibronectin is released into the vagina when mechanical damage or damage caused by inflammation occurs to the membranes. If the test is negative, it is 98 per cent certain that you are not in labour, despite other evidence such as the presence of regular contractions. Preliminary results seem to indicate that a positive test provides less useful information but the importance of a negative result cannot be overstated, especially in early pregnancy when a decision as to whether to transfer you to a distant unit with advanced special care facilities may need to be taken.

If you are more than 35 weeks pregnant, it is unlikely that anyone will make an attempt to prevent labour beyond perhaps a bit of bed rest. Your baby is likely to be perfectly fine and it doesn't make sense to try and stop labour at this stage. Other situations in which labour will not be halted include haemorrhage, an infection within the womb (chorioamnionitis), placenta praevia and severe pre-eclampsia.

Causes

There are some very obvious causes of premature delivery. The first group all involve some decrease in the amount of bloodflow available to the womb and include placental abruption, placenta praevia, diabetes, renal disease, cardio-vascular disease and pre-eclampsia. The second group are also familiar and involve overdistention of the womb, including multiple birth, abnormally shaped womb and too much amniotic fluid (polyhydramnios). Abdominal trauma (accident or surgery), incompetent cervix, retained IUD, infections and maternal acute illness (e.g. appendicitis, pneumonia, fever) may result in premature delivery, as will premature rupture of the membranes (see pages 213–15).

These are what you might call the obvious causes. There are also a whole raft of 'predisposing factors', of which the first and single most important is a previous premature birth. Evidently if you have had a premature birth because of a condition which is not likely to repeat itself (like placenta praevia, road accident or an illness), you have a very high chance of having a normal term delivery next time around. The reported risk of recurrent pre-term labour varies between 17 to 50 per cent but is generally quoted as about 35 per cent. The risk increases with each subsequent pre-term birth and may be as high as 70 per cent following two or more pre-term deliveries.

Other predisposing factors include smoking (which is very

strongly associated not only with premature delivery but babies of reduced weight), drug use (especially cocaine), emotional stress, two or more children at home, long tiring daily journeys to work, being an unsupported mother, teenage pregnancy, poor weight gain, heavy work, lack of antenatal care and living in poverty. I should point out at this stage what 'predisposing factors' means. It does not mean that if this is your third baby you are automatically a candidate for a premature baby. Rather like risk factors for pregnancy outcome, there is a balance, with negative factors on one side and positive on the others – the fact that you are healthy, well fed and well housed, for instance, will far outweigh minor negative factors. Finally, it is also likely that gestation is genetically programmed to some extent and that gestation length is therefore an inherited characteristic, with members of the same family having roughly similar gestation lengths.

You may have read all the above and found that none of it applies to you. You are not alone – about 50 per cent of premature labour is termed idiopathic, a medical weasel word which basically means the same as the curious DBK notation you sometimes come across in medical records: it actually stands for 'don't bloody know', and that's about the strength of it. Prematurity affects a minority of pregnancies, yet it accounts for nearly three-quarters of all baby deaths. Although the outlook for premature babies is infinitely better than twenty years ago, the rate of prematurity has remained pretty much constant. This is partly because, it has to be said, the process of labour itself is not yet fully understood. It's rather like a manufacturing production line in which you know what the end product is, you know what parts are needed to make it, but you don't know the precise sequence of production and most importantly, you have no idea where the 'on' switch is that starts the whole thing up.

Premature Rupture of the Membranes

In some pregnancies, for reasons that are not entirely clear, and in the absence of any contractions, the sac holding the baby breaks, causing the amniotic fluid to start leaking out into the vagina. There is some evidence that abnormal membranes, which literally have weak spots, may be the cause, and once again infection is also implicated, as is multiple pregnancy for obvious reasons. You will see this written as PROM in notes (premature rupture of the membranes) or as PPROM, pre-term premature rupture of the membranes. PROM occurs in up to 15 per cent of pregnancies, with about a fifth of these taking place before 36 weeks.

Very often women find it difficult to tell whether their waters have broken in this way. There may not be a sudden rush, but a slow trickle of fluid, which sometimes leads women, particularly if it is early in pregnancy, to suspect incontinence rather than a leak of amniotic fluid. I have to come clean here and say that when my waters broke, three weeks ahead of time, despite working at the time for Birthright, I rang the obstetrician in a panic. 'What shall I do?' I said. 'I think I'm incontinent.'

Amniotic fluid is alkaline and hospitals have special test papers which stain blue in the presence of amniotic fluid. You might also distinguish it by the white or greasy particles in it. You yourself can test whether it is amniotic fluid: if you dab your finger in it, then wipe your finger across a piece of glass and allow it to dry, you will see a beautiful ferny pattern.

Amniotic fluid has many functions. It provides a pool in which the baby can move, grow and develop symmetrically, without any pressure on its delicate tissues. It also helps maintain an even temperature and contains an antibacterial substance.

Most women with ruptured membranes at or close to term, say from 36 weeks on, will go into labour soon after the rupture has occurred – 70 per cent will deliver within 24 hours, and 90 per cent within 48 hours. About 5 per cent will not go into labour and remain undelivered after 7 days. Some hospitals remain keen to induce women as soon as possible when the waters have broken in this way, because of the risk of infection; but the best evidence suggests that a policy of induction of labour following rupture of the membranes at or very near term exposes the mother to a higher risk of caesarean section and maternal infection as well as to a longer and probably less comfortable labour. However, to minimise the risk of infection, once your waters have broken you should not make love and you should also pay scrupulous attention to personal hygiene, particularly after using the loo.

If you suspect you are leaking amniotic fluid, it is vital that you tell someone about it. Depending on your circumstances (stage of pregnancy, etc.), you may be admitted to hospital. You may have an internal examination, although some hospitals prefer not to do this at all. A sterile speculum may be used – a digital vaginal examination is usually not undertaken since infection might be introduced to the womb. And infection is the major concern. If the membranes rupture before 26–28 weeks, the baby has an increased risk of a number of problems, the most important of which is the likelihood of developing breathing problems. This is because the baby requires amniotic fluid, not only for its lungs to mature, but also to practise breathing movements.

What to do when a woman's waters break very early is one of the most controversial subjects in obstetrics. Many hospitals prefer a policy of 'expectant management' consisting of bed rest and continuous observation for signs of infection, like raised temperature or increased heart rate, or any other indication that the baby is in trouble. The thinking behind this practice is that the longer the baby can have in the womb, the less likely it is to have breathing problems at birth. About 50 per cent of women with pre-term rupture of the membranes will deliver within a week, although a rough rule of thumb is that the more premature the baby, the longer the time period before spontaneous labour begins following rupture of the membranes. Whilst it is possible that the leakage will stop and the fluid reaccumulate, this is the exception, but sometimes quite a bit of fluid remains and if a few extra weeks can be eked out, by continuous bed rest, then the baby is likely to fare better when it is eventually born. At very early stages of pregnancy it has to be said that major loss of amniotic fluid is an ominous sign. Without sufficient fluid, the chances of the baby having lungs healthy enough to survive are slim indeed. One of the most effective forms of care is also one of the simplest – checking that there are facilities available to care for a very tiny baby on site, or transferring the mother to a centre that does have the expertise and facilities to ensure that the baby has the best possible chance of survival when it is born.

You might think that, in these situations, drugs which halt labour would be a good idea, especially if contractions have not yet started, but these do not seem to be of much benefit in preventing the onset of labour. Antibiotics, however, are often administered routinely, in addition to corticosteroids – drugs which help to mature the baby's lungs rapidly. If you have signs of an active infection, a more aggressive regime of antibiotics will be started and delivery effected as soon as possible.

Stopping Premature Labour

If your waters have not broken, and you are in an early stage of premature labour, a variety of drugs can be used in an attempt to arrest labour. None of them is universally successful and to be effective enough to suppress the strong contractions of the womb they may have side effects on the mother or the baby, some of which may be undesirable. They are called tocolytic drugs and can only be used in cases of uncomplicated premature labour (that is where there are no other problems like maternal diabetes or heart disease). They fall into two broad groups: the first is beta-mimetics, the best known of which is called ritodrine (trade name: Yutopar). Other names you may hear are salbutamol and terbutaline. About a third of women will experience palpitations with these drugs, together with restlessness and agitation. A particular concern is the possibility of an accumulation of fluid on the woman's lungs, called pulmonary oedema. There are also alterations to some physiological processes like control of sugars and potassium levels. The drugs are infused at first, then, if labour is inhibited and side effects are minimal, the infusion is gradually scaled down until finally the drug can be given by mouth.

The other major group of labour-inhibiting drugs are prostaglandin synthesis inhibitors, of which the best known is indomethacin. These drugs are not generally used as a first-line treatment, although they are more powerful inhibitors of contractions than beta-mimetics. This is because they have not yet been fully evaluated. The concern with these drugs is that one of the jobs of prostaglandins during pregnancy is to keep the circulation of the baby in its aqualung mode (obtaining air via the mother), and that a drug which has anti-prostaglandin properties might, in theory, cause the baby's circulation to switch to air-breathing mode before birth. Early trials were reassuring on this point; nevertheless, the drug tends to be used only for short periods of time.

For many years neat alcohol was recommended for inhibiting labour. This always seemed curious to me, since a great folklore exists about the use of alcohol to do precisely the opposite, i.e. set women off in labour, and as an agent for inducing abortions. It has now fallen out of favour because, although there is some evidence that it works, the side effects are unacceptable. In any case, if you're going to go for broke on the alcohol front, having it out of a warm plastic drip bag without the ice and lemon doesn't seem at all fair.

Being in Labour Too Soon

Going into labour too soon can be an alarming experience, partly because a million questions run through your mind about the health of your baby. If you had hoped for a natural birth you may feel rather alarmed, not only because of the amount of equipment in the room, but also by the number of medical staff in the room, most of them completely unknown to you, who have come to look after the baby as soon as it is born. In addition you will almost certainly find yourself wired up to all sorts of monitors because of the need to keep a very close eye both on the progress of the labour and particularly on the health of your baby. You may have very mixed feelings; on the one hand you want everything possible in the way of high tech medicine to be available for your baby, but on the other hand you may be wailing inside that this wasn't how you wanted it to be. Choice about childbirth options in these situations is unfortunately very often dictated not by parental wishes but by that baby of yours.

Just because your baby is likely to be smaller than others doesn't mean that the labour will be less painful. There is, however, a more restricted range of pain relief options available to women in premature delivery because of the need to avoid narcotics or sedatives which depress the baby's breathing. Epidurals are usually recommended.

Some obstetricians think that premature babies, particularly those lying in a breech position (remember that very often babies don't turn into the head-down position until relatively late in pregnancy, so that a much higher proportion of premature babies are in the breech position than at term), should be delivered by caesarean. There simply isn't a consensus of opinion on this and research does not make a strong case either way. You will, however, find that measures are taken to protect the baby's delicate head as much as possible, such as an episiotomy and perhaps even forceps.

Most parents find premature births pretty traumatic – not necessarily because of the birth itself, but because the situation escalates so quickly that they feel totally out of control and helpless. Parents often speak of the birth of their premature baby as having a dream-like quality, as if the whole thing were happening to someone else. Shock is a major emotion for many parents, as is guilt. Even though you may know that the reason for prematurity is completely outside your control, you will still manage to manoeuvre yourself into believing that you were somehow the cause of your baby's predicament. You may find yourself subject to extraordinary swings of mood, from elation to despair and back again. And worst of all, you may be very frightened.

When the baby is born you may be able to cuddle it straightaway, but the baby may need immediate attention at birth, perhaps then going into a resuscitation trolley before going swiftly to the special care unit. Very often a photograph will be taken so that at least you have something with you when your baby is away from you. Your baby may look very different to the baby you were expecting, with a large bony head and a very skinny body. The skin looks almost transparent and may be covered with soft, downy hair. Premature babies are often rather frog-like in the way they lie, with arms and legs out to the side and knees bent. Some parents describe their first glimpse of their premature baby as like 'meeting an alien'. The baby is not of course horrific to look at, yet this baby may be so far away from the image of the baby you thought you would have that there is a sense that it isn't yours. Sometimes parents are reluctant to touch or hold the baby and it may take some time before you come to terms with feelings like this.

Your baby may be given surfactant treatment at birth to help prevent the type of breathing problem known as respiratory distress syndrome. Surfactants are chemicals that reduce surface tension – a good household example is washing up liquid – and they play an important role in our lungs. Were it not for surfactants, our lungs would stick together when we breathe out. If you inflate a wet plastic bag you'll see what I mean: when the air leaves the bag, the sides stick together. Hard as you try, you'll find it very difficult even to open the bag, let alone inflate it, but if you add a drop or two of washing up liquid you won't have a problem. Babies born prematurely do not yet have sufficient surfactant in their lungs. All babies must clear the fluid in their lungs and replace it with air when they take their first big breath, but because premature babies do not have enough surfactant their lungs don't inflate properly and remain waterlogged. Respiratory distress with grunting and rapid breathing may then occur. This is called respiratory distress syndrome (RDS) or hyaline membrane disease (HMD). Not just premature babies suffer from this condition; it also occurs in babies born to diabetic mothers, twins, and in some babies born after an emergency caesarean.

Once the waters break, a baby's lungs mature rapidly and within forty-eight hours will contain a greatly increased quantity of surfactant, even if the waters have broken prematurely. Giving the mother corticosteroid drugs at least forty-eight hours in advance of labour will help mature the lungs and help prevent RDS. If neither of these things has happened, the next preventive step is to administer an artificial surfactant to the baby soon after delivery. Some surfactants are prepared from animal lungs and are called 'natural' surfactants because they closely resemble the real thing. Synthetic surfactants have become increasingly sophisticated recently and one, Exosurf, is now in regular use. All surfactants are extremely expensive, costing as much as £1,000 per treatment course.

There is conclusive proof that surfactant treatment reduces both the severity and mortality of RDS and that it also reduces the risk of pneumothorax (in which the lung collapses following rupture). Curiously, some of the complications associated with RDS, such as brain haemorrhage and long-term lung disease, are not reduced. About 10 per cent of babies will not respond to surfactant treatment, although this might be partly because they do not have RDS in the first place but have another lung problem, such as pneumonia, instead.

Special Care

Of course not all babies in special care are premature; some have conditions that may require surgery or have other health problems following the birth. When you first visit a special care baby unit (SCBU), it's the equipment you see, not the babies, who seem completely overwhelmed by machinery. Normally the unit is divided into three areas: a maximum intensive care section, a high dependency section, and a nursery for babies that are almost ready to go home.

It can be very frightening when you first see your baby 'wired up' and it helps to find out what each of the wires and bits and pieces actually does.

BREATHING

There are usually three sticky pads attached to wires which are placed on the baby's chest, and these are to monitor the baby's heartbeat and the rate and depth of breathing. If your baby is breathing on her own, you may find that there is an alarm device on the mattress instead of these. For many babies with breathing problems, treatment with oxygen will be all that is necessary. Oxygen-rich air is supplied to the incubator from an air-oxygen blender to a seethrough headbox which stabilises oxygen levels around the baby's head. But if the baby's condition gets worse, a machine may have to do her breathing for her until her lungs have matured or healed.

The ventilator is usually box-shaped with various bits of tubing attached to it, and on a trolley so that it can be moved around. One lot of tubes goes to a supply of air and oxygen (usually located on the wall behind) and another set of tubes takes these gases to the baby. A small tube, an endotracheal tube, is passed through the baby's nose or mouth into its windpipe and then fixed to a collar which can be attached to the baby's face with tape. This endotracheal tube is then attached to the ventilator. Having a tube in your windpipe isn't very pleasant and many babies become agitated and restless. Pain relieving and sedative drugs may be infused through a catheter on the baby's wrist and a splint (very often of green gauze) holds this in place. Despite the fact that a baby is on a ventilator because he cannot breathe regularly and the machine is pushing air and oxygen under pressure into the baby's lungs between 20 and 40 times a minute, sometimes the baby will attempt to take breaths of his own. These may go against the ventilator and cause the baby's condition to worsen. Modern ventilators, however, have become increasingly sophisticated and some now incorporate a triggered ventilation system. This means that the baby can breathe some breaths on his own, but if his breath is not enough to expand the lungs fully the ventilator is triggered to give a breath to the baby.

You will normally find two further electrodes on the baby at around tummy level; one monitors temperature, the other the amount of oxygen the baby has in his blood. This latter job may be done by a tube threaded through the baby's umbilicus which can also be used to take blood samples and blood pressure measurements, in the light of which the settings on the ventilator can be adjusted so the baby gets just the right amount of oxygen. If a baby is being ventilated, it is unable to clear phlegm from its lungs by itself, so from time to time a nurse will place a fine suction tube down the endotracheal tube to suck out the secretions.

You may be concerned about oxygen therapy because of the risk of blindness. The pop singer Stevie Wonder is just one person who became blind as a result of oxygen therapy because of prematurity, and this was certainly a big problem in the fifties and sixties. However, the risks are now very well understood, and providing that oxygen levels are kept within well defined limits during the time the baby might get this condition (up until he would have reached the equivalent of about 32–34 weeks gestation), the disease (retinopathy of prematurity) is exceptionally rare.

FEEDING

Many babies in special care are too little to digest milk or even to suck properly (this latter skill would normally develop at around the 32 week stage) and may have problems in co-ordinating sucking and swallowing. Fluids and nutrients may have to be given direct into the baby's bloodstream, and once the baby is mature enough to digest milk it will be fed through a tube down the back of the nose into the stomach. Breast milk is the best milk for special care babies and nurses on the unit will show you how to express milk, but even so you may find that the baby's feeds have to be topped up with a special formula milk designed for premature babies. After about 34 weeks, the baby will start sucking. However, breast feeding a premature baby can be an exhausting process because they are often very sleepy until they are about 38 weeks old and it may take all sorts of subterfuge, from foot flicking, toe tickling and the like, to nappy changing immediately before a feed, to stimulate them enough to keep sucking. Only trial and error will show you what works best for your baby but it can be a very frustrating time. The NCT have a leaflet about breast feeding premature babies and the La Leche League may also be able to help you. If the baby isn't sucking very much and has to be topped up with nasal tube feeds, you will need to express frequently, as without regular stimulation your milk supply may begin to fade.

TEMPERATURE

Tiny babies are not able to regulate their body temperature as we do, and they lose heat very quickly. Normal babies conserve heat by curling into a ball, but premature babies adopt the 'frog' position in which they expose a large body surface area which loses heat rapidly. Many of the incubators have radiant heaters to minimise potential heat loss, but these can potentially cause a different set of problems because, for the very same reasons that the babies lose heat so quickly, they also lose a lot of water and dehydrate in high temperature conditions and overheat. Some cots have humidifiers. Babies will usually wear bonnets or hats (the head is the greatest source of heat loss) and you must remember to be aware of temperature and its potential effect on your baby when you are handling him.

Changing and Other Procedures

During the day, the medical staff in the unit will carry out routine procedures and checks on the baby such as taking a blood sample and changing the nappy. Some parents want to be present at these times, others don't. Don't feel shy about asking to be present.

CLOTHES

You may have a whole drawerful of baby clothes back home, waiting for a 7 lb baby. The clothes that seemed so minute when you bought them will now seem gigantic, completely swamping your little thing of 4 lbs, and your baby will literally have nothing to wear. Alternatively, you may not even have thought about baby clothes yet. Don't despair; SCBUs usually have their own supply or run a clothes library. In addition, both Mothercare and Boots have tiny versions of standard terry stretchsuits and BLISS (see Appendix I) have a leaflet called 'Products for babies in SCBUs' listing specialist suppliers of tiny clothes, nappies and other items.

COMMUNICATING

Care of special babies is very complex. Most staff are very good at explaining, in simple language, what they are doing and what needs to be done. Neonatal paediatricians take great pains to discuss what care is appropriate and to involve parents in decisions about care. SCBUs are stressful places and staff understand what you're going through, so never be afraid to let go or to ask for help, support or advice.

BEING WITH YOUR BABY

One of the major findings of the last twenty years has been the recognition of the psychological problems that can be caused by separation of a baby from his mother. This is even more true of the premature baby; and premature babies that do not have contact with their mothers do not thrive as well. Touching, handling and stroking your baby has an immensely beneficial effect and skin-to-skin contact is the recommended way to cuddle your baby, so don't be surprised if you are asked to slip your baby down your shirt, for some skin-to-skin contact. Even if your baby's eyes are closed he will still know you are there from the sound of your voice and touch. Singing or reading to your baby will help both you and him. It's important too that brothers and sisters are allowed to see the baby, as well as grandparents, and most SCBUs are very easy about visiting hours for close relatives, although they may insist on masks if your other children have colds or coughs.

If you have a very sick premature baby, you may find it difficult to bond with your baby. You may find that you are on emotional auto-pilot, unable to think or feel consistently. Part of you wants to surround the baby with love and affection but part holds back, for fear of being hurt should things worsen and the baby not make it. You may feel angry, guilty, but above all responsible and at the same time helpless. Even when your baby is out of immediate danger he may still seem very fragile, but that wall full of photos of chunky toddlers inevitably present in every SCBU is what you need to concentrate on. They grow up to be big healthy louts that will drive you mad, leave the towels all over the bathroom floor and eat you out of house and home just like other babies.

You may feel very worried about your baby's long-term future, but the statistics, not to mention flesh-and-blood examples like Isaac Newton and Sir Winston Churchill who were both premature are reassuring. Only one in ten premature babies suffers any form of handicap from being born too early and the proportion of babies who come through the experience completely healthy is growing all the time. You may find that your baby crawls or walks a little later than other babies – you just have to be a bit more patient. On the intellectual front, development is usually perfectly normal, although some tasks that require concentration and shape recognition, such as complex jigsaws, may take more effort if your baby was born before 34 weeks. I have to say that I have come across more than my fair share of premature babies and most of them are possessed of demonic energy and have very strong personalities. In fact, my general experience is that premature babies go on to rule the roost with a vengeance. You have been warned.

Preventing Premature Labour

For many years American organisations such as the March of Dimes have had an extensive teaching programme aimed at prevention of pre-term labour. The American rate of pre-term labour is higher than in Britain, largely as a result of the lethal combination of restricted access to health care and extreme poverty and deprivation, particularly in big cities. No such comparable programme exists in Britain and you may be uncomfortably aware as you read some of the recommendations of the gap between your well educated, well fed and well housed life and the lifestyle of those for whom the programme was principally designed. Nevertheless, there are some useful points which you might find helpful.

Stop smoking.

Avoid substance or alcohol abuse.

Eat well consistently (poor weight gain and prematurity are linked). Try not to go for long periods without eating as this can provoke prostaglandin release (prostaglandins are involved in the labour process).

Drink at least a cupful of water every waking hour and avoid drinks containing caffeine (which promotes water loss from the body). Taking adequate fluids decreases the release of antidiuretic hormone (the hormone involved in water balance) and increases the bloodflow to the womb. Drinking frequently will also reduce the likelihood of urinary tract infections.

Try to prevent urinary tract or vaginal infections by drinking adequate fluid, keeping the perineal area clean, avoiding scented bath salts (see the recommendations in Chapter 6 on how to avoid common pregnancy problems) and also limit sexual contacts to one person. If there is any evidence of an infection – e.g. burning or stinging when urinating, or discharge, report it immediately.

Try to empty the bladder at least once every two waking hours as a full bladder can stimulate the uterus to contract and also increase the likelihood of infection.

Try to plan your day to reduce activities that are tiring and to include at least one rest period to increase bloodflow to the uterus. This also decreases risk of prostaglandin release. If you have a stressful life, try and learn relaxation techniques, or include regular exercise such as swimming or walking which decrease fatigue and stress.

Be aware of the warning signs of early labour, such as period-like abdominal cramps, dull backache, a change in vaginal discharge, or diarrhoea, and know what a contraction feels like. It is a tightening sensation that does not have to be painful.

If you have any of the above warning signs, empty your bladder, lie down on your left side and drink two to three cups of water. If the warning signs do not go away after the hour of rest, or if you are experiencing more than four contractions an hour, call your doctor. Incidentally most pregnant women experience tightenings of the womb, but those that are not at risk of premature labour will have three or less an hour.

Particularly towards the end of pregnancy, if you have a single partner, and always if you have multiple partners, use a condom, as semen contains prostaglandins which may precipitate labour.

Avoid twiddling your nipples (seriously!) as it stimulates the production of oxytocin.

Finally, back to a favourite hobby horse: almost all pregnancies are stressful in some way or another; life's like that. Families have to be cared for, the mortgage has to be paid and there is of course that thing all women seem to subject themselves to – moving house or having building work done – when pregnant. So it's all too easy to find stress in your life when you're desperately trying to discover why you had a premature baby and of course to blame yourself. Don't. You haven't done anything more than a hundred other women just like you, all of whom had babies at term. You drew the short straw and that's all there is to it. You've got a special baby, but with special care and affection he's more than likely to do just fine.

16

Breast Feeding

Most women have already made up their minds whether they are going to breast feed or not well before their delivery. The proportion who decide to breast feed during pregnancy is actually quite large (nearly two-thirds) but there is a dramatic fall off soon after birth with only about 20 per cent of mothers continuing breast feeding after the first week or so. You don't need me to tell you what the benefits of breast feeding are – you've been told them a million times: best for baby, best for you, convenient, hygienic – so why is it that so many women give up? Well, here's the truth – and this comes from someone who breast fed her children until two and four years of age: in the first couple of weeks, breast feeding can be hell. Your nipples are sore, nobody else can do it, you seem to be permanently leaking and attached to a baby, and you may well begin to wonder why you ever thought this was a good idea. What is more, there is a conspiracy, even amongst carers, which prevents you breast feeding properly – by which I mean staff offering supplementary feeds, unhelpful advice and even samples of formula. Persevere, however, with breast feeding and it is simply bliss.

But first, those of you who have decided not to breast feed. You will find that within three or so days of birth your milk comes in. You may go from being a modestly endowed woman to one that could model for a top-shelf magazine any day of the week. If you have always had the sort of breasts that run for cover under your armpits, post-birth breasts can be a complete revelation – and a bit of a nightmare. I, the sort of woman who could have a bus driven down her cleavage, had a bosom so big I could hold a pencil between my breasts six inches from my chest. If you are not breast feeding, what on earth do you do with such things?

Two of the most commonly offered 'prescriptions' are to restrict fluid intake or to bind the breasts tightly with a cot sheet, neither of which has been scientifically validated but which, with centuries of experience behind them, both seem to work. Cot sheets are probably more painful in the short term, but work better in the long term than drugs. Bromoergocriptine is the drug of choice and has no serious adverse effects, although about 5 per cent of women will feel nauseous. Most hospitals do not offer drugs routinely but see how you are getting on first, as these drugs can be expensive. Whatever you do, if you are not going to breast feed don't be tempted to express milk in an effort to reduce the pressure as it will only fool your breasts into believing that more milk is required.

How do you succeed with breast feeding? It seems to me that the dogma that pervades bottle feeding (every four hours, etc.) has invaded breast feeding as well. There is a great deal of very poor information – one of the greatest new myths is that if you don't put the baby to the breast immediately after birth the chances of successful feeding diminish. Babies are not all ready to feed at the same time, and if you need proof that I am right about this, remember that in some cultures, breast feeding is delayed until milk proper, as opposed to colostrum, comes in, with no diminution of breast feeding success. The really important time is the first feed, whenever that is. You need to be quiet, perhaps with your partner there as well, and relaxed.

The key to successful breast feeding is position, position and position. The trouble is that we are not equipped with under-bosom wing mirrors, which is what you really need to check that your baby is positioned properly. It is easier for other people to see than you, which is why having your partner there can help, and one of the advantages of being in hospital is that you will see other women breast feeding, something you may not have had close access to in the past, which will help you understand what is required.

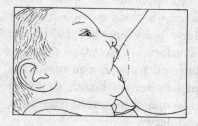

Baby incorrectly
positioned at breast.

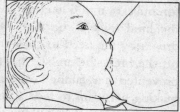

Baby correctly
positioned at breast.

Before I get on to the mechanism of feeding, a word about nipple preparation. There is a hysteria about nipples needing to be 'conditioned'; various solutions, from light scrubbing with a nail brush, application of creams, even surgical spirit, have been advocated for use in the months prior to birth. There is no evidence that any of them work. If the baby is positioned correctly there should be no friction on your breast. Instead, the baby does it for you. She fashions a teat out of not just the nipple but the surrounding breast tissue as well by the suction created in the mouth. The nipple only accounts for about a third of the teat created by the baby and it is the action of the baby's lower jaw on the underside of the breast tissue that is critical in transferring milk from the breast to the baby. Thus the baby needs to look as if it has a good bit of breast inside its mouth, not just the nipple. If your baby is correctly positioned, you should feel no pain and you shouldn't get a lot of nipple soreness.

Unfortunately, many of the breast feeding practices advocated by well meaning staff follow the old 'must toughen up the tits to avoid soreness' route which cause the very thing they are aiming to prevent. For instance, you may be told to restrict your baby's access to the breast, allowing her only a couple of minutes per side at first and building this up gradually. There are several components to milk – the foremilk, is, if you like, the low calorie thirst quencher, whilst the hind milk is the high calorie gold-top stuff. Babies are driven by the need to consume calories. If you take the baby off the breast before she has finished feeding, you may have prevented her taking sufficient calories on board, therefore making her want to feed again sooner than would have been the case had she finished her feed herself.

Of course you may offer your baby feeds when she wants, and for as long as she wants, only to discover that far from being a contented happy babe she is still wanting to be fed on the hour, every hour. This can be absolutely the worst moment in breast feeding. After a while babies sort out their own daily rhythm. It may not be exactly what you had in mind, but it is a pattern of sorts. But at first they are all over the place and may indeed want to feed all the time, which can be incredibly wearing. I think it is particularly hard on women who have had careers beforehand, because suddenly you find yourself completely trapped by the demands of this tiny thing, which doesn't even have the grace at this stage to smile at you for all your trouble. Suddenly, stretching before you, is the enormity of the change in your situation. You may have felt that you could take a baby in your stride and fit it in with everything else, but here you are, unable even to get dressed by lunchtime or complete the smallest task because of this wailing baby that refuses to be satisfied by your very best efforts. It will sort itself out, I promise, and feeding every hour doesn't continue.

Another thing that may shock you is the length of time that it takes to give a baby a breast feed. Reading the books, you'd think that ten minutes would do the trick. Think again, although some babies feed quickly, others feed incredibly slowly, especially if they are sleepy, but also if they are born by caesarean section, are having special care, are jaundiced, etc. It will take all your efforts to keep the little darling awake – my husband resorted to flicking our baby's toes with a teatowel. At the other end of the spectrum are the babies who are so damned interested in everything else that they continually stop and crane round before resuming feeding. Thus it may be that, if your baby is feeding very frequently, by the time you have changed her, taken off your shirt that the baby has been sick on, and sorted yourself out, it is time for another feed. This struggle is made worse by the remarks of well meaning mothers, aunts and neighbours, who will mutter under their breath that in their day you fed the baby every four hours and that was that – as if they had not a spot of bother from their babies. Well, they did; but they've forgotten.

You might think, if you have a baby that is feeding very often, that you have not got enough milk. Only a very small number of women, perhaps 5 per cent, genuinely do not have enough milk, and it is therefore unlikely that this is your problem. Carers used to attach great significance to weighing the baby before and after a feed in order to find out how much milk the baby had taken, the idea being that if too little was taken supplements could be given, and if too much was taken breast feeding could be restricted. There is no justification for this whatsoever; as you will realise, restricting breast feeding simply means a very hungry baby and a smaller supply of milk, whilst supplementing is a pretty surefire way to bring breast feeding to a halt. Such measurements are usually very inaccurate, and as babies vary immensely in how much milk they need the practice is flawed from start to finish. Incidentally, one of the comments about breast feeding you may hear most often from older women who bottle fed is, 'How do you know how much you're feeding them?', because in their day feeding was ruled in ounces and how many had been given at each feed. Again, quantity is immaterial; what you want to know is, 'Does the baby seem well and happy?'

At the very beginning of breast feeding, while you are still in hospital, one of those lovely midwives who always seem able to soothe your fretful baby instantly and whom you would really like to pack in your luggage and take home with you, may offer to give you a bit of rest by feeding the baby with formula. Women whose early breast feeding is supplemented by formula feeds are five times more likely to give up, so don't be tempted.

Babies do not need supplements of water, glucose or formula. Even when it is very hot, babies have no need for large volumes of fluid other than that supplied by the breast, and it is a myth that extra night-time feeds won't hurt, because this is when prolactin (the hormone that controls milk letdown) is released. Encouragement with breast feeding is far more important to you at this stage than offering a supplement crutch, however welcome it may seem. Whilst your midwife, La Leche League counsellor or health visitor may be crucial, particularly in advising you about positioning the baby during feeding (latching on), what may be equally vital is the friendship of other mothers in the same boat as you, who are probably all thinking exactly the same – why on earth did I ever think this was a good idea? One of the great advantages of the National Childbirth Trust is the way in which it fosters friendships amongst pregnant women attending their classes which are continued after the babies are born. It is all too easy to feel that you are on your own, particularly if you are a professional woman who, because she is not normally home during the day, has few friends in the immediate area.

I said breast feeding suffered from dogma. There are babies who do not thrive at the breast, despite their mothers' best efforts and the best efforts of those who care for them. If your baby is failing to thrive, isn't putting on weight, then health professionals should recognise this, and should not insist on your pursuing breast feeding when it plainly isn't working. Having said this, the vast majority of breast feeding problems can be resolved with good positioning, unrestricted access to the breast for the baby and practical and emotional support, but if nothing seems to work, for heaven's sake take to bottle feeding and feel positive about it. You are doing the best for your baby, not failing.

Recognising whether there isn't enough milk is not that easy. If you find you are constantly feeding, your nipples are sore and your baby's motions are few, dark green and hard with very few wet nappies, then you might need help. If the position at the breast is right and you are feeding frequently and not restricting feeding in any way, you might need more rest (an afternoon rest does wonders for the evening milk supply) or a better diet yourself. If you are taking medicines (antihistamines are a particular culprit) they might affect your supply. Finally there are drugs which can be given to increase supply – these include metoclopramide and sulpiride.

There are various minor niggles about breast feeding. One is the leaking breast syndrome. This varies from woman to woman, and in most it seems to settle down after a month or so. However, for a while you will find that whenever your baby cries, or just before a feed, or from the other breast when feeding, you will leak like crazy. And I don't know what the physiology of sitting in a hot bath involves, but expect a milk shower from both breasts when you sit in the tub. Breast pad technology has improved tremendously of late; nevertheless you will find yourself getting through millions of them in the early months, so lay in a good supply. It also helps to be aware of the type of clothes that are most affected by spreading milk stains, and to avoid these if you have to do something respectable. If you have sore nipples, and you leak a lot, it could be that you are irritating the nipples by letting them wallow in a wet mess of a plastic-backed breast pad. A bit of air to your nipples at every feed is probably the best solution. A frequently recommended solution to leaking is to sprinkle cold water on the areola (the area around the nipple) as this is supposed to tighten up the muscles. I have yet to be convinced by this.

Another stain factor that no one seems to mention in books but which is obvious the moment you see most new mothers is that babies are sick on you. If you are very well supplied with milk, you may find that when the baby first feeds, it gushes out all over the place, with the baby constantly spluttering and coughing as she struggles to cope. These babies often take in a great deal of air with the feed and, although they feed quickly, reward you by being sick afterwards. You can try expressing a bit of milk first, as this might help with the flow, and sitting the baby in a more upright position, but otherwise there is nothing much you can do, apart from draping a terry nappy or muslin square over your shoulder. In fact, if anybody ever offers you terry nappies accept them, even though you intend to use disposables. They are brilliant wipers, sick-blotters and general all-round indispensable baby items. Some babies are just naturally sicky – it doesn't mean that they are ill, that's the way they are. Incidentally, breast-fed babies' sick is a lot nicer than bottle-fed babies' sick: the first smells milky, the second like sick.

My first baby was loudly sick after every feed. When he was two weeks old, I had to go to an editorial meeting at *Woman* magazine. The editor was a childless woman, not at home with babies. The meeting went on and on and gradually the carrycot in the corner came to life. I knew that a feed would have to take place. Making myself as invisible as possible in the corner, I prayed for Owen to be sick quietly. He was, but as I was leaning forward on the chair it splatted straight into my shoe. Unable to clear out my shoe in full view of the editorial team, I just had to squelch my way home.

Another problem is lack of suitable places for breast feeding when you are out and about. I have fed my babies on trains, planes and in a collection of sordid public lavatories, there being no other place to feed them. You don't actually have to display your breasts to the world when you feed; it can be done very discreetly. Nevertheless, I would feel embarrassed about feeding in front of those people whom it might offend. It's not that I'm embarrassed myself, just embarrassed for the seventeen-year-old lad trying desperately to look the other way – and I think you have to be sensitive about this. But when this would mean feeding a baby in a stinking British Rail loo, I told myself firmly that I was adding to this lad's life experience and ignored his discomfiture. Be bold.

I would be lying if I said that women whose babies were correctly latched on did not have nipple soreness. They do, although not to the same degree as those whose babies have their mother's nipples like a terrier has a bone. Sometimes this is because the breast is so engorged with milk (the old Chesty Morgan trip on day 3 or 4) that the baby finds it difficult to latch on. Engorgement is quite tricky to deal with. The temptation is to express like mad, but although a bit of expressing helps, doing too much doesn't. I was well supplied with milk for my first baby, but for my second my body went into complete overdrive. Lying on my front was out of the question; so was a bra, although a hammock would have done, and it all got wildly out of control. Even my obstetrician took one look at me and said very firmly, 'Vivienne, we'll have to do something about those.' My midwife suggested a compress of cabbage leaves. My husband duly visited the greengrocer but all that happened was that my jumper was stuffed not just with a pair of enormous leaking tits but a lot of partially cooked greenery too. Binding with a sheet did the trick in the end and I still had enough milk for an army of babies. If engorgement does not respond, then there are some drugs, oral proteolytic enzymes, that can be very effective. Two homeopathic remedies, belladonna and bryonia, are said to work well.

Rubbing your nipples with some of the milk at the end of the feed (the hindmilk) will keep your nipples supple, but otherwise, although there are a great many potions, cooled boiled water is as good as anything. However, if a potion makes you feel better, the homeopathic remedy calendula (marigold) in cream form is probably the first one to try. The important thing is to seek help from your midwife as quickly as possible, rather than letting things get out of hand. Some people swear by nipple shields, although they tend to prolong the agony in my view because feeds take so much longer, but you may get on with them fine. If you are dreadfully sore, express for a couple of feeds, thereby resting your breasts, rather than give up altogether.

There are a number of other tips to avoid soreness. Don't pull the baby off the breast – most cling on like limpets and breaking such a substantial suction force is a sure recipe for maternal damage and infant annoyance. Put your little finger in her mouth and release the suction that way. Make sure that you put her to the breast gently, supporting her with a cushion if need be, and supporting your breast with your hand if you find it helps. Change position frequently so that if there is a sore bit, it isn't being pressed on continuously. It may help to sleep without a bra so that you get a bit of air to your nipples, or even to sit for five minutes in the sun with your breasts exposed, if it is summer. If you are having problems with blockages, when part of your breast is lumpy, reddish or feels bruised, seek immediate help, because mastitis may follow, which is rotten.

If you are well supplied with milk in these early stages, and are planning to go back to work, or want someone else to look after your baby for a bit, then express milk while you have it in quantity and freeze it. The things you have to remember about expressing are cleanliness and hygiene. Wash your hands before you start to express, sterilise the breast pump if you are using one and make sure the container you put the milk in is also sterile. Boots now sell special freezer bags for breast milk. You don't need a breast pump, although it can take the effort out of expressing.

If you are going back to work, you may get yourself in a panic about expressing. You may try introducing the odd bottle of formula, reasoning that this will do no harm when breast feeding is so well established and you need to go out without baby. It is at this stage that you may discover that your baby wants nothing to do with a bottle. You might try someone else giving the bottle; after all, why should your baby accept a bottle from you when he can smell the real thing is on hand? You might also consider swapping teats; some, particularly in the Pur orthodontic range, are more natural to the baby than others. Alternatively, and this is well worth knowing, try getting your baby to take one of those double-handed sucking cups containing juice or boiled water as early as possible because they will sometimes take to those cups when they won't touch a bottle. This approach means that a lunchtime feed can be substituted by solids and fluid from a cup by about 3–4 months. This will ensure that you can go on breast feeding morning, late afternoon and evening and soon cut down to two breast feeds or so, leaving a good part of the day when you can go out without your baby if you have to work.

Although it is fine to take the mini (progestogen only) pill when breast feeding, you shouldn't be taking the ordinary pill as it will affect your milk supply, as well as going into the breast milk. You should be aware that your breast milk is a physiological fluid, and what gets into the rest of you will get into breast milk. This includes alcohol, nicotine, some (but by no means all) medicines and the breakdown products of food. You may find that your baby is particularly sensitive or colicky after you have had certain types of food. Brassicas of any sort, very spicy food and orange juice are the culprits I most often hear mentioned but it varies enormously from one baby to another and what may affect one may have no effect on another. Some mothers say that their babies are rather jumpy and restless if they drink a lot of coffee, and certainly caffeine can pass into breast milk so be aware of this.

Whilst the old wives' tale about having to drink milk if you want to breast feed is false, the premise that a good diet is important to breast feeding is very true. It's not just your milk that needs a good diet at this stage – you may find that you are rather tired, and you should make an effort to eat properly, with quality meals spread throughout the day, rather than, for instance, just one main meal in the evening. You may find that you are quite thirsty, particularly when you are actually feeding, but advice to drink more fluids than thirst dictates in order to make sufficient milk is unwarranted and will just leave you feeling bloated.

The main message that I want to get across about breast feeding is do not despair and give up in those early days. It can be grim, but I would be failing you if I didn't tell you how wonderful breast feeding can be as the baby grows. If breast feeding is not your thing, then I don't think you should be made to feel guilty about it – providing that you don't influence other women trying breast feeding to give up. Let them work it out themselves.

17

After the Birth

'Nobody ever told me how long it takes to get over the baby, physically and mentally.'

'I never knew how tiring it would be afterwards or how sore I'd be.'

'I wish I'd known about the physical highs and lows in the first two weeks after the birth, and the swinging from heaven to hell hourly.'

'I wish I'd let people help more after the birth – I really regret not doing so now.'

'I wish I'd known how long it would take my body to get back to normal.'

'Nobody ever said that there could be problems after the birth.'

'Afterpains – they were a complete shock.'

'I never knew that bleeding could be so heavy afterwards.'

'I wish I'd known that sex would be such a disaster.'

'No matter how awful the pregnancy and birth are, babies are worth it all, and your body will return to normal. After all, most people go back for a second go!'

*'From being the centre of attention, I suddenly found
that I was invisible. I was sore, dog tired and all anyone
wanted to do was coo at the baby. I kept wanting to
scream "What about me?".'*

*'I kept saying to my mum that my life wouldn't change.
Boy – was I in for a shock.'*

Having a baby is just the start, as so many women pointed out
in the survey. Yet, curiously, almost everyone except the
parents regard it as the end, a job well done, congratulations all
round, thank you and goodnight. In general, pregnancy books
are part of this conspiracy. Very little is said about 'afterwards',
although it is a time when you desperately need information,
help, and above all support. Even if your delivery was
uncomplicated, the combined effects of no sleep, trauma and
high emotion will have exacted their toll on your body. You
will not be looking your very best. If *Hello!* wants a picture of
you and your baby, be sure not to choose the day after
delivery.

*'If only I'd known that I would not get up after delivery
with a flat stomach, looking wonderful.'*

The first revelation – for revelations these are – is that you still
look pregnant after the birth. This may lead you into some
dreadful, both-feet-straight-in gaffes when you, complete with
bump, arrive at the hospital to have your baby. 'When is your
baby due?' is a reasonable opening gambit with a woman you
meet on the ward – providing you are not asking someone
who delivered her baby three days earlier. If your *bon mot*
happens to coincide with that rush of hormones known as the
baby blues, there may well be tears before bedtime.

'I wish I'd known my stomach would look like a deflated cream puff.'

Sadly, without that baby and fluid in there, your stomach doesn't have quite the proud prominence it had before. It just looks like a horrible flabby old lump. If you have this sort of stomach after delivery, it is sod's law that the next bed in the ward will be occupied by a woman who came in, delivered, and a few hours later put on her jeans – yes, her jeans – before going home. She will have done this in full view of the rest of the ward, you can be sure. Content yourself with believing that these are not her normal Armani size 8s but a pair of size 16 specials bought for the purpose.

There is no point despairing about the state of your flab at this stage. There's a mile-long queue of bodily parts to despair over – your stomach can wait. Comfort yourself with the thought that actually some of your flab is to do with fluid retention (the if-in-doubt-blame-it-on-the-fluid ruse). Actually this is true, particularly if you have had an epidural, with its concurrent drip; if you have had any infusion containing oxytocin (Syntocinon) whose anti-diuretic properties will have caused fluid retention during its use; or if you had a lot of oedema before delivery.

You may also find yourself sweating profusely – not because the hospital is hot, although they always are, but because your body is attempting to get rid of this fluid. Sweating may continue for some weeks, especially at night. You can help speed up the process of fluid elimination by drinking drinks which have a diuretic effect, such as coffee and tea. Be warned, however, that the last thing you want if you have desperately sore parts is to be peeing every five minutes. One further piece of advice about fluid intake postpartum; you may be told that you need lots to drink if you are to have enough milk. There is absolutely no scientific evidence that increased fluid intake will result in improved lactation, so please don't feel you have to. Just drink if you are thirsty.

You may have been one of those walking wounded who managed to bounce out of the delivery suite and back to the bed. You may, on the other hand, be one of those who had to be delivered to your bed in a wheelchair. Let me tell you that even the walking wounded will have felt as if a six-ton weight was about to fall out through their vaginas. Even if you are one of the 30 per cent who escaped the need for stitches (revelation number two – 70 per cent of women in the developed world have damage to the perineum that requires stitching), your perineum will still feel as if it has been kicked. The situation isn't helped by having to wear industrial grade sanitary towels, which make you walk like a cowboy.

You may hit the pillow and immediately fall asleep. Many women are on a complete 'high' and find it impossible to rest or sleep. All I can remember doing is staring at my baby in amazement – here he was at last. Some are consumed with hunger, since most haven't eaten much, if anything, for twenty-four hours. Hospitals run a tight ship with regard to mealtimes and if you have missed the evening meal, you may not be fed until breakfast. Whilst some hospitals have tea-and-toast facilities, many do not. By this time, like as not, all the public hospital catering outlets are shut. At this moment you may bless your mum for sending you off with a packet of chocolate biscuits in your luggage. Although I am making light of this, there is a serious point. Having something to eat is often a fast way of making you feel a lot better, as some of what you feel is simply the motoring equivalent of having run out of petrol and 'running on fumes'.

'I'd had no food for forty-eight hours. I was so weak it frightened me.'

Problems with Passing Water

Before you settle down to sleep, make sure that you have had a pee. It won't be as easy as you think (revelation number three – you may find it very difficult indeed to pass urine after delivery). Bladder control is effected by several sets of muscles – one set is under your control, which is why you can stop mid-stream if required. Another set, the detrusor muscles, support and surround the bladder. Bound up in them are the muscle fibres of the urethra (the tube that leads from the bladder to the outside). When the detrusor muscles contract, the sling of muscle relaxes, allowing the bladder neck to widen into a funnel shape so that the urine flows into the urethra. Both sensation and the detrusor function of the bladder are reduced by the residual effect of epidural anaesthesia, by the administration of sedatives and analgesic drugs, and of course by the pain, bruising and swelling caused by trauma to the perineum. Over-extending the bladder with urine happens all too easily. Once it has happened a vicious cycle ensues, in which bladder sensation and detrusor function are further impaired. It may take several weeks to recover from this. In addition, having a pool of stagnant urine in the bladder predisposes to bacterial infection. Women having epidurals will have urine removed via a catheter to avoid this happening (they are of course unaware that their bladders are full).

It will take every trick in the book at first to persuade your bladder to part with its load of urine but, for the reason I have outlined, it is very important. One of the best tricks is to run a tap or trickle water, but many gynaecologists swear by immersing your hands in a basin of cold water. An injection of a drug, carbachol, may be used if these home remedies fail. What makes it even harder is that you may be required to perform this impossible task on a bed pan. If you possibly can, walk to the loo as this in itself will help. Nursing staff are alert to the possibility of urinary distension and will normally pester you for an account of your waterworkings. If you haven't passed urine within six hours of delivery, and nobody has asked, tell someone. A catheter may be required, which sounds a lot grimmer than it is. Besides, a brief flirtation with a catheter is, let me assure you, a lot better than prolonged acquaintance with a sulky bladder. If you have a lot of stitches, you may find that urine stings like mad. Take a jug of water with you to sluice yourself down, or fill the bidet with water and pee in that. Urine is sterile so it will not harm you. Peeing as the bath water is draining out is another tip which may help.

Incontinence

'One piece of advice? Keep doing your pelvic floor exercises – you'll thank me when you're fifty!'

Some degree of urinary incontinence in the last months of pregnancy is very common indeed, mostly because pregnancy hormones relax the bladder supports. You may have noticed this, particularly if you leaked when coughing or sneezing (stress incontinence). This is not a pattern for life. However, it may not resolve as quickly as you might wish following delivery: 25 per cent of newly delivered mothers will find that they still have some degree of urinary incontinence following birth. For the vast majority, this will resolve. About 1 in 10 women will have a residual problem. Don't ignore it. As I have indicated, it is very common indeed, not at all something to be ashamed of, and very treatable.

In case you are worried that 'treatable' means surgery, it doesn't. Although surgery is an option for some forms of incontinence, scrupulous attention to your pelvic floor exercises will usually do the trick. You will read again and again of the importance of undertaking pelvic floor exercises, both for healing and for future sexual function – the prevention of incontinence is top of the list. Your midwife will instruct you how to do pelvic floor exercises. If you find them difficult, there are a system of traded, weighted cones which can be used in the vagina each day, which do much the same thing. The address from which you can obtain these is given in Appendix I. You can try these exercises out on your partner whilst lovemaking; if you are doing them right, it should give him (and hopefully you as well) quite a thrill. Suddenly they don't seem so bad after all.

Bleeding After Delivery

'I wish someone had told me how much you bleed afterwards.'

Many women's experience of periods will have been coloured by the fact that they were on the pill for much of their lives. If you have always had light periods, the bleeding and discharge following childbirth, technically called lochia, may frighten you as it can be quite heavy. If you are at all anxious, tell someone. The blood comes from several sources, such as tears, but most importantly from the wound left in your womb when the placenta came away. The inside of your womb has pretty remarkable powers of regeneration – remember it goes from the womb equivalent of parquet floor to luxuriant shag pile during the course of every month – so it will soon heal. In addition remember that your placenta was very well supplied with blood vessels. Were it not for the fact that your womb contracts after delivery, squeezing these blood vessels shut, they would continue to bleed and you would very soon bleed to death.

At first the blood loss is bright red. After three days or so, it becomes brown, then pinkish yellow. It has a characteristic sweetish odour. If it starts to have an offensive smell, or if bleeding gets heavier not lighter, please tell someone, as it may be the first sign of an infection or that not all the placenta has come away. Such bleeding may continue for as long as six weeks, or for as little as two.

Some practicalities for a moment. You will be given a supply of the industrial grade sanitary towels I described earlier – usually about a day's worth. After that, you're on your own. Bring more maternity pads than you are ever likely to need as asking your partner to pop out to the chemist and buy more seems to induce faint hysteria in men. There is no need these days for those little belts as most towels are sticky-backed. No matter how often you change them, leaks will still conspire to wreck your knickers. With maternity wards, it is strictly a take-out laundry service. In other words, it means either washing your knickers yourself in hospital or sending them home for laundry with your partner or mum. You can do without this sort of hassle. Get in a supply of disposable paper knickers (the NCT do some, or use the men's sort from Boots which seem designed for real people, unlike the women's sort which are designed only for dolls or Kate Moss). Alternatively, save up your passion-killer pregnancy knickers (see my section on thrush) and chuck them away after use. This may be the first time in your life that you have used sanitary towels; although tampons may be what you prefer, they should not be used in the post–partum period because of the danger of infection.

Afterpains

'I wish I'd known about the period-type pains you can have in the early weeks and that they're normal.'

The midwives will check every day on the position of your womb, which will, over the next ten days or so, return to its original position, somewhere just above your pubic hairline. The faster it does this, the less likely it is that you will haemorrhage, because contraction is shutting off those blood vessels tight. The womb will need to contract for some time after delivery in order to achieve this feat. You may notice this particularly when you are breast feeding, when the combination of hormones that stimulate your milk also makes your womb contract sharply. This can hurt. In fact, these 'afterpains' can be almost as painful as labour for a few women.

This is no time for heroics. Strong analgesics, particularly if taken half an hour or so before breast feeding, are in order. Paracetamol is the analgesic of choice as it will not affect the baby if you are breast feeding. You may notice that following these afterpains you have a bright red blood loss. You might think that afterpains were a reason for not breast feeding. In fact you are doing yourself a favour by breast feeding because anything that helps the womb shrink will help reduce the duration of bleeding. In any case, painful afterpains only last a few days, although you may be aware of slight crampy pains whenever you feed for several weeks. These afterpains are usually worse with second and subsequent babies, because your womb, having been stretched before, has to work harder to get itself back into shape.

On the first day you may pass clots of blood. This is normal. However, the passage of clots should not last more than twenty-four hours. If you pass a particularly large and alarming clot, call a midwife and let her quickly check that it is a genuine blood clot, rather than a bit of retained placenta. Once again sod's law will be at work – the clot will slither into the loo and you will be torn between being squeamish about retrieving it, and being public-spirited about telling the midwife. The halfway house is to let someone else retrieve the blithering thing, but you would be wise to say something.

For ten days your pulse rate, temperature and blood pressure will be measured daily, with at least four measurements of each in the first twenty-four hours. The reasons for this are in part related to the bleeding. A combination of slight fever and prolongation of red lochia much beyond the third or fourth day may indicate an infection, or that a small piece of the placenta has been left behind in the womb. If this is the case, going to theatre to have the womb properly emptied under general anaesthetic will be necessary, as these little bits of placenta are potent sources of bleeding. A drop in blood pressure and a rise in pulse rate might also indicate the type of blood loss which, if it is sufficiently heavy to affect your vital signs, should be investigated.

Excessive Bleeding

There are two terms you will hear used which describe excessive bleeding following childbirth. One is primary postpartum haemorrhage. It may occur between the delivery of the baby and that of the placenta, or it may occur after the placenta has been expelled. About 2 in every 100 women will have an excessive early blood loss. It is clear that many of the women in our survey who had dramatic haemorrhages were, despite the transfusions and the dashes to theatre, unaware that their life was threatened. Whilst they knew that they were bleeding, they seemed not to be aware of the extent of the bleeding, partly because they couldn't see it (which helps), but partly because they had their baby and that was all that mattered. Everything else was an anti-climax and of no importance. Their partners, on the other hand, were all too well aware of what was going on and were terrified. Post-partum haemorrhage is not as significant a cause of maternal death as it used to be, but it still constitutes a full scale emergency, which in itself is a cause of alarm to the mother and her partner. Nearly 70 per cent of deaths due to haemorrhage are caused by post-partum haemorrhage.

In 90 per cent of cases of post-partum haemorrhage, the cause is that the uterus has failed to contract properly (uterine atony). There are several predisposing factors: having a womb that has been over-distended, for instance because of multiple pregnancy or too much amniotic fluid (hydramnios); or having a womb that cannot contract down properly because of the presence of large fibroids or a retained placenta. Other factors include instrumental deliveries and prolonged labours, especially of a big baby, ending in a forceps delivery or section. Occasionally injudicious yanking on the cord before the placenta has separated can be the cause.

The doctor or midwife will attempt to make the womb contract by massaging it internally and by giving an injection of a potent womb-contracting drug (oxytocin and/or ergometrine) into a vein or muscle. If this fails, an injection of a hormone-like substance called a prostaglandin may have to be put directly into the womb muscle. Depending on the amount of blood loss, a transfusion may be required or other fluid drips. Your vital signs will be monitored very closely. Blood loss causes a reduction in blood pressure and prolonged low blood pressure has to be avoided because it might otherwise result in heart, kidney or liver failure, hence the requirement for transfusion.

'I never thought that mothers could be ill after a birth and might end up needing a D & C.'

Secondary post-partum haemorrhage describes bleeding that is far less dramatic and dangerous than primary haemorrhage, and which occurs after the first twenty-four hours following delivery and up to six weeks following childbirth. Such bleeding can still have serious effects and may be caused either by infection or by pieces of the placenta remaining in the womb. Very often these factors occur together. Blood loss can either be sudden, profuse haemorrhaging or, perhaps more commonly, increasing rather than decreasing loss of lochia. Your womb may not have diminished in size as it should have and the neck of the womb may not have shut tight. Because infection is very common in these circumstances, expect the need for tests to establish exactly what bacterium is responsible for it and to be put onto antibiotics. An ultrasound scan may also be used to help identify pieces of placenta retained in the womb. You might think, in your misery, that it is complete medical incompetence – I mean, how could they not know that some of the placenta has been left behind? It isn't, unfortunately, as simple as this. Although the placenta is checked very carefully when it is delivered, the fact that bits are missing is sometimes not as obvious as you might think, particularly if the placenta is in poor condition.

Once the antibiotics you are taking have started to have an

effect in controlling infection, and your temperature (if you have one) has started to decrease, you will need to go back to hospital. Under a general anaesthetic your womb will be emptied. Depending on how poorly you are, this might be just a day procedure. You will be able to take your baby with you. If you are breast feeding, it shouldn't interfere too much.

Your First Period

'My first period was worse than the labour.'

This seems to be a deeply neglected subject, judging from the survey results. If you are not breast feeding, your first period may return before the six week postnatal examination. In the normal way, the release of an egg and the accompanying alteration in hormone levels is the signal for the womb to begin shedding its lining. However, ovulation has not occurred, and as a result the womb lining has just built up and up – ever since delivery. When you do have your first period (which could be several months after the birth if you are breast feeding), it may be abnormally heavy, prolonged and often very painful. The amount of blood loss can be a bit alarming. You may also pass large clots. In fact, menstrual blood does not clot – it contains potent anti-clotting agents. The 'clots' you see are actually large balls of red blood cells, formed because you are bleeding so quickly that your menstrual blood is running out of its anti-clotting factors. Although this is all a bit worrying, it is not usually a sign that there is anything wrong. This is not a lifelong pattern of menstruation for the future – just a one-off. However, if the blood loss is very severe you should go to your GP who may prescribe a hormone preparation which will control the bleeding. An oral contraceptive may be appropriate, especially if this is what you were planning to use anyway.

'I wish he'd worn a condom – babies eleven months apart nearly killed me.'

One word about contraception. About six hours after the birth, at a time when lifelong celibacy seems a pretty attractive proposition, someone with a horribly cheery smile will loiter at the bottom of your bed and ask what sort of contraception you intend using. I have no evidence whatsoever to support this, but I have always thought that these good people work on a commission basis, rather like double-glazing salesmen, with points going to the one who can sign up most mothers for contraception in a week. How else could they persist, when it is plain that sex is unlikely to be on the agenda in the next six weeks, let alone the next six hours? Mind you, there are exceptions. I was once sitting next to a man at a dinner. I remarked that his children were very close in age. 'Well,' he said, 'if you've got a private room at Queen Charlotte's you might as well use it.' It takes all sorts.

Stitches

'I really worried about having stitches. And I did have them. In fact, they weren't a problem at all. Nobody told me about piles, the pain of which I attributed to stitches.'

As I have said, 70 per cent of women in the Western world will have some sort of repair following delivery. Thus it is more likely than not that you will have stitches. It is clear from the survey that stitches were a source of great pain and distress in some women. Having said that, just because you have a few stitches doesn't necessarily mean that it will hurt.

The problem with stitches is that things tend to get worse before they get better. If you don't know this in advance you will, by the third or fourth day, begin to panic and think that either the wound is infected or, worse, that someone with the needlework skills of a five-year-old has sewn you up far too tight. Let's deal with infection first.

You have an open wound in your womb, and you have several acres of bruised and battered flesh. You are heaven on legs to a bacterium with an eye to the main chance. Infection is unpleasant, debilitating and, in the main, avoidable. Unfortunately maternity wards, particularly their bathrooms, are rarely as clean as they ought to be. So the ball is almost entirely in your court, and you should be scrupulous about personal hygiene following delivery. If you are at home, of course, the bacteria are more likely to be your own and to do you less harm. Nevertheless, some of the measures below will still apply to you.

You may feel that sloshing antiseptics about, particularly in the bath, is the best way to avoid infection. In fact the use of strong antiseptics will delay healing and may cause irritation. Here are some practical, sometimes obvious but nevertheless essential tips.

Wash your hands after using the loo. Wash your hands before and after changing a soiled towel and change your towel frequently. Do not use a shared roller towel to dry your hands, but paper towels. If you have washed your genital area, do not dry it with a towel, even if it is your own. For preference, pat it dry with paper towels or tissues which can then be thrown away. If your stitches are very sore, briefly drying the area with a hairdryer set on the cool setting is helpful, but get your partner to bring your own dryer in and do not share it with anyone. Do not overdo this, as overdrying can delay healing; in fact many people would not recommend the use of hairdryers.

If you have a bath, or use a bidet, make sure that you clean it before use, even if the previous occupant has cleaned it. Avoid using the sort of bidets that have fountain showers (even at home). When using the loo, sit well back so that your vulva does not touch the seat. Wipe the seat if you can with an alcohol wipe. If the staff seem reluctant to offer you these, insist. Do not use loo rolls if they have been sitting on the floor.

If you are using an ice pack or rubber ring, rinse through a new J cloth and use it as a cover. Throw it away after use. A pack of J cloths accompanied me in my luggage when I arrived in hospital to deliver my second baby, simply because first time around there were never any cloths with which to clean the baths, which were invariably filthy. If the baths are just too sordid, showers are more hygienic. I have some sympathy with hospitals. Maternity wards are busy busy places and on the go twenty-four hours a day. Cleaning is in general a daytime, nine-to-five, Monday to Friday job. To some extent, women have to be responsible for their own hygiene. Given my activities with the Vim and the J cloths, I think they were quite keen to keep me in for the week.

Having avoided infecting your wounds, here's how to cope with the pain and general discomfort. As I said, stitches often get worse before they get better. The body's healing process goes through a stage in which fluid accumulates at the wound site, particularly on the cut edges of skin. The swelling that this causes means that stitches bite tighter for a while, but this terrible feeling of tightness will wear off as the swelling subsides. After a week you should be feeling a lot better.

You may feel easier soaking in a bath, but oversoaking is

not a good idea. Having salt in the bath is not harmful but
there is no evidence that it speeds healing either. Avoid using
bubble bath and too much soap, particularly if it is highly
perfumed. Whilst you are in the bath, you might gingerly
explore your perineum – it may feel horribly lumpy. Shocked
by this revelation, your mind then begins to work overtime:
how you'll never be the same again, how your husband will
desert you. The only (vaguely) analagous situation I can think
of is when you have an injury in your mouth – perhaps a
jagged edge on a tooth, or an ulcer. To your exploring
tongue the wound seems immense, but if you looked in a
mirror you would quickly see that it was relatively minor. It is
much the same here. If you can bear it, look at your perineum
with a hand mirror. It may look pretty bruised, but the
wound and stitches may not be half as awful as you had
imagined.

> *'I was worried my stitches wouldn't heal properly and I'd
> never be the same again. They did of course, and I am,
> but I never shared this worry with anyone.'*

There are various potions you can use to aid healing and
deaden pain. Ice packs numb the pain, but although they may
help a little in reducing swelling, they will not promote long-
term healing. This is because as surface blood vessels contract
in response to the cold, blood is diverted away from the area.
You need a good blood supply to promote healing. If you are
using ice packs (a 1 lb pack of petits pois is made for the
purpose), wrap them – a paper dishcloth is ideal (otherwise
you'd end up with a freeze burn as well as sore bits) – and
dispose of the wrapping between use.

Several local anaesthetics are available, in gel, spray, cream
or foam formulations. Lignocaine gel seems to be the first

choice. Although you might think that, with all that inflammation, creams containing hydrocortisone would be effective, steroids impair wound healing and should not be used. Many people claim witch hazel to be very effective, although a trial showed it to be no more effective than tap water. If you are a witch hazel believer, soak a pad with it and apply it directly to the bruised areas.

Other home remedies include honey, which has antiseptic and healing properties. To say that it is sticky, however, is an understatement and you may well end up cursing me for even suggesting it as you attempt to remove the sticky patches from bed linen, clothing and your husband's pyjamas. Of the homeopathic remedies, arnica has much to recommend it, either taken orally or used as a cream. Calendula cream is also healing, but none of these remedies has been subjected to proper trials.

What has been subjected to trials and is known to work is something else you may curse me for. Having had a baby, you may not feel that you have any muscles left below the waist, but if you do pelvic floor exercises as soon after delivery as possible not only will you experience less pain, but healing will be quicker. This has much to do with the increase in bloodflow stimulated by pelvic floor exercises. If you can bear it, four or so tightenings about every fifteen minutes should help a great deal. Although you may feel that reclining on the bed is much the best option, being as mobile as possible will also help healing, again by stimulating bloodflow.

On the increased bloodflow basis, the use of ultrasound or pulsed electromagnetic energy (both of which you may find offered by the hospital physiotherapists) is increasing, although it is not clear whether either offers as much benefit as claimed.

Finally, the low tech solution. Sitting on a rubber ring (a child's swimming ring will do) can be enormously helpful, although you shouldn't use them for too long as they put undue strain on your pelvic floor.

Having exhausted ice, witch hazel, rubber rings and the like, what next? Paracetamol or ibuprofen (Neurofen) are the painkilling drugs of choice. Very little of either is carried with breast milk, and both are effective. Codeine-containing preparations (e.g. Codis) are stronger analgesics but should be avoided because they tend to make you constipated, which is the last thing you need right now. Aspirin should also be avoided because it prolongs bleeding time (it thins the blood) and is transmitted to the breast fed baby. If you hurt in hospital, ask for painkillers when you need them.

Finally a note of empowerment. Of course stitches can hurt, of course they can be uncomfortable, but this should fade fairly quickly. If after ten days or so you are still experiencing discomfort and pain, tell someone. Do not think that you have to wait until your six week check before you can moan. If you get the 'what do you expect, you've had a baby' routine, do not meekly accept this. Continue to tell your doctor and, if necessary, ask him to make an appointment for you to go back to your consultant. Of all the telephone calls I get about problems following delivery, the tales of continued pain and miserable sex are the ones that get my goat most, mostly because these women's pleas for help have been ignored. Women should not, and ought not, to accept pain as part of the aftermath of childbearing. If sex is painful, tell someone. Despite what we think in our darkest, most exhausted moments, sex is not an optional extra denied to parents. Good sex is fundamental to our self-esteem and self-worth. Flabby stomachs and stretch marks are one thing – this is quite another. Do not accept it.

Having said all that, there are some complications of stitches which are worth noting here. Trapped surface cells beneath the skin can occasionally result in the formation of a cyst, called an inclusion or epidermoid cyst, either with episiotomies or stitched tears.

'A cyst formed where I'd had an episiotomy stitched. Sex was impossible for nine months till it went. I went to the doctors three times before anything was done.'

For very painful scar tissue, smooth glass dilators may be helpful. These are passed into the vagina several times each morning and evening, starting with the largest tolerable and continuing with small increases in size until there is no pain. Sometimes a raised area, which may be frond-like, and which is red and bleeds easily, forms. This is so-called granulation tissue, which is caused as a result of an over-enthusiastic healing process by the body, sometimes in response to irritation by stitches, or as a response to low grade infection. This can be removed easily by cautery.

Part of the underlying reason why women are reluctant to complain is that they fear having to return to hospital to be restitched. It may not have to come to this – but even if it does, from all the tales I have been told, it is infinitely preferable to struggling on in misery for months and months.

On Stitches, Sex and Rock 'n' Roll

'I wish I'd known that other people's babies are all crying and waking up in the middle of the night too.'

In those desperate days when you first get home, when you are exhausted, leaking and debilitated, when your hair has lost its pregnancy sheen and your baby is at its most demanding and impossible, you consider yourself to be an asexual being. Sex appals. For a start you are too tired – who wants to make love; all you want to do is crash out and sleep? For another thing, who in their right mind would find this flabby, leaking mess attractive? And then of course it's out of the question because it will be too painful and awful. And the stitches might burst and you'll be so stretched inside that you'll be completely unrecognisable to your partner. Stop right there.

Of course you may not feel like it right now. But good sex has never been just about penetration. When you are feeling completely wrecked, there is nothing nicer than to be cuddled and held, to be close, comforted and comfortable with the person you love. Relaxing into this sort of cuddling, without any pressure for lovemaking, does wonders for you. It's important for your partner too. Remember that it isn't just you who has been through a life-altering experience. Your partner went through much the same sort of emotional swings – elation, acute anxiety, exhaustion – and now this; a completely changed role, that of a father. He now has to share you with a baby and he may find it difficult to adjust to this. He needs to feel that he is still as important to you and that you still love and value him as much as you ever did. It is very easy to focus all of you on the baby and leave nothing for him; if he cares – and most of them do – he will understand at first, then be hurt, and finally resent it.

Some women who breast feed find that their libido increases. A postgraduate obstetric textbook I read claimed that high levels of oxytocin (the hormone involved in the milk letdown response) meant that women got to orgasm more quickly. I am personally of the opinion that this is male fantasy. Very many women find that their libido goes into hibernation for a while following delivery. Another problem for the breast feeding mother is that leaking breasts offer a constant reminder of motherhood rather than sexuality.

The important point about resuming sex is not to rush. When you first start to be aroused, stick to oral sex or mutual masturbation. Enjoy giving each other pleasure and enjoy feeling aroused and sexy (despite your leaking breasts and flab). When you feel ready for penetrative sex, be very tentative at first, and don't expect the earth to move. Treat it like your first time, and you may well be rewarded with one of the most tender and special experiences of your life. If you are breast feeding, your vagina will be dryer than usual. Even with lots of foreplay, you may still not be as lubricated as you would normally be. I don't need to tell you the difference between making love when you are fully aroused and well lubricated and making love when you are unaroused and rather dry; the latter can be sore and unpleasant, and that's with fully functioning bits, rather than a vagina that has been violently assaulted by a baby in recent weeks. Being tense doesn't help your general level of lubrication either.

The first time you make love again is especially important to you both. If it's a disaster, it will colour your views of sex for quite some time. You will also, after so long without it, have to think about contraception. Some women ovulate within three weeks of delivery. Even women who are breast feeding can ovulate as early as two months after delivery. Believe me, nobody who has babies just a year apart recommends it, so be warned. If you are breast feeding, barrier methods of contraception are preferable because oestrogens in the pill affect milk production. The progestogen–only pill (the so-called mini-pill) can however be used, as very little progestogen gets through to the breast milk (the equivalent of one tablet received by the baby over 1,000 days of lactation). If you want to use the cap, you will need to get a new one (at your six week check), and not rely on the one you had before you got pregnant, as your internal shape will have changed. An IUD (coil) is a good contraceptive to choose if you have completed your family, and the postnatal check at six weeks is an ideal time to fit it.

In terms of lubrication, you need all the help you can get. If you are using a condom, you might try a lubricated variety. Replens is a vaginal moisturiser (available over the counter in pharmacies) which lubricates the vagina for three or four days at a time. It may also help you feel more comfortable if you are suffering from excessive dryness. Senselle and KY jelly (available from the chemist) are lubricants which can be used at the time of lovemaking. Senselle is more discreet and probably preferable; KY jelly definitely needs a bit of warming up first – it's a bit gloopy otherwise. Rather than you putting the lubrication on your partner, as part of foreplay get him to put it around the entrance of your vagina. You can tell him the bits that hurt still and it will help make him sympathetic to your needs. It will also reassure him that basically you are still the same as you were – remember, he was the one at the business end during the delivery and his imagination is probably running riot. One of the unspoken worries that came out of our survey was the 'vagina as a sack' one. You were concerned that the vagina would be so stretched that you would be unrecognisable to your partner. The man that says he can tell just by the feel of lovemaking whether a woman has had a baby or not is a lying toad. The vagina is very stretchy and, whilst other bits of you take longer to return to normal, your vagina is back to its normal size within about a week. Put this worry out of your mind.

> 'You can forget spontaneity. It's strictly when you can, i.e. when the baby's asleep.'

You might find you have to adjust your positions the first time. Side-by-side positions, or you being on top where you can more easily control penetration are probably best. Even if the bit where you had your stitches has stopped hurting most of the time, it will probably be quite a long time before it is completely pain-free when lovemaking. Be gentle and take it slowly. If it really hurts, be honest and say so. Don't just lie there gritting your teeth wishing it could be over quickly. This is a sure recipe for that most unpleasant of vicious circles: fearing lovemaking because of pain, becoming very tense, lovemaking being awful because you are so knotted up and then wanting to avoid it altogether.

There are several other must-know things to do with post-partum sex. Unless you are advised otherwise, most stitches will have healed within about three weeks. Gentle penetration will not tear your wounds asunder. Although penetration may be a bit painful at first, the very act of penetration stretches the tissues. The more you stretch them, the less likely they are to hurt. This may sound completely perverse, but actually, if pain is very severe, treatment involves the woman using a series of glass dilators, each bigger than the other, over a series of weeks, to stretch the vagina. It is usually very successful treatment. If penetration is very sore at first, ask your partner to use his fingers – it will help stretch you, be less worrying possibly than full intercourse, and hopefully turn you on as well. Finally, pelvic floor exercises will help, as I said before, to promote healing, tighten things up and enhance sexual response, so don't give up on them.

When is it normal to resume sex? What's normal hair colour? There is no right answer to this one. Amongst our survey respondents, just 27 per cent had resumed sex by six weeks; for the vast majority, sex wasn't on the agenda until much later. For a significant minority (5 per cent), sex wasn't resumed for a year or more. You may feel very anxious about the effect that no sex, or very unsatisfactory sex, is having on your partner. More than one respondent said that she thought her partner would stray if sex wasn't resumed quickly. As I said before, sex is about more than just penetration. It may take you both a long time, depending on the circumstances of your delivery and of your situation, before you even start to fancy each other again, let alone make love. It helps if you both understand this beforehand. If this is how it is, and it is something that you have both acknowledged and discussed, and you are still sharing touches and caresses, although not indulging in penetrative sex, don't let others' opinions on how they think your sex life should be worry you both. Sexual feelings will return; you just need the space and time – and, it has to be said, most importantly the opportunity – for it to happen.

If you want an illustration as to how this might be achieved, here is my personal recipe. There is something ever so erotic and forbidden about making love on a weekday afternoon (you can tell I'm a working mother, can't you!). Book yourselves into a posh hotel for the afternoon, leaving baby firmly behind. Being pampered and feeling naughty may just do the trick (and don't forget the KY either).

A final word on sex. I firmly contend that babies are born with ESB – extra-sensory bonking – powers. They have an unerring ability to wake up and shriek the place down the minute either of you takes a foot off the floor, or worse, do a complete number on you just as you reach orgasm, completely wrecking your day. You might laugh about it once. When it gets to be a habit, as it will, it becomes a source of tension. You can never really get into the swing of things, because you are waiting for the baby to cry. You may also feel unable to be completely abandoned in your lovemaking because you feel constrained by the presence of the baby, especially if its cot is in your room. Suddenly, the baby is an alien. It's asleep but it knows what you are doing. You sense waves of disapproval.

What if it's damaging for babies to have their parents bonking in the same room – even when they're asleep? It's madness of course, but sometimes it just doesn't feel right and there's no getting away from it. After all, we all know that our parents only had sex twice, once for us and once for our brother, and never did it otherwise; and you are a parent now.

Sane parents plan that Granny comes to lunch, and disappears (having done the washing up of course) with baby in pram to some far distant park afterwards. The problem with this ploy (I've tried it, believe me) is that when you actually have two hours without your baby, your libido completely disappears and all you want to do is either rush round catching up with chores you can't do with the baby about, or slump in front of the telly and sleep. At least do it in each other's arms, for heaven's sake.

> *'Just leave the housework – it's the one thing you can be sure will still be there tomorrow.'*

There is sex beyond childbirth, I promise. And it can be as good as you want to make it.

Haematomas and Piles

I am aware as I write that the title alone of this section is enough to make most people skip a page or two. But piles and vulval varicose veins were amongst the top five 'secret worries' of our survey respondents. They are unpleasant, can be very painful but are also unmentionable. After all, tell someone about having sore stitches and they'll offer tea and sympathy. You don't even want to talk about piles, yet they may be causing you just as much pain.

Varicose veins of the vulva can be a source of considerable worry as well as discomfort. They often appear in the latter months of pregnancy. Women assume the worst and think that they will burst under the strain during labour. They don't. It is often said that ruptured vulval varicosities are the cause of vulval haematomas (localised collections of blood). This is not usually the case at all. It is far more likely that bleeding from a tear or an episiotomy had not been effectively controlled before stitching. As a result, a pool of blood accumulates. This may cause acute pain in the perineum, with the woman complaining of feeling unwell, looking pale and feeling giddy. Some haematomas can contain quite large amounts of blood, and transfusion may be necessary, after which the haematoma is dealt with and the source of bleeding stopped, usually under general anaesthetic. Interestingly, haematomas are more common in women who deliver on birthing stools.

You may have had piles before delivery. They may be worse afterwards, or alternatively you may experience piles for the first time. Try pushing back protruding piles, using a little Vaseline on your finger. Once up the rectum, they shouldn't be quite as painful. If they protrude when you've passed a stool, push them up again. All the general self-help measures for piles described in Chapter 6, such as avoiding constipation, using soft loo paper, avoiding squatting, etc., should be followed. There are a number of anaesthetic creams, e.g. Anusol, available which may help. If your piles are really uncomfortable don't endure them in silence; tell your GP who can offer you industrial strength pile preparations, and who can also reassure you that you are quite normal. Piles are very common, and probably those most likely to get them are pregnant or newly delivered women.

Constipation

The British have an obsession with the workings of the bowel. In some hospitals, concern about your urinary functions may be completely eclipsed by an almost nanny-like 'have you been yet?' mentality. In fact, some hospitals don't allow you out until 'you've been'. The truth is that, particularly if you are on a twenty-four-hour discharge, you may not want to go. Often the bowels will have been cleared before the birth, and the combination of slower gut motility and very little food intake may mean that you actually won't need to open your bowels. When you do, you may feel the urge to bear down. You may panic and think that, of all things, this may be what bursts all your stitches. Don't panic. This is unlikely in the extreme. If you are really worried, gently hold a clean pad against your stitches, and push upwards whilst you bear down.

There is such an obsession about bowel opening that laxatives, stool softeners and enemas may be offered routinely (without any real justification). If you are constipated, bulk-forming laxatives are less likely to cause unpleasant cramps and diarrhoea than are irritant laxatives. It seems to me that constipation in hospital follows the same pattern as the sort of constipation seen in young schoolchildren: you hang on until you can sit down in the quiet privacy of your own home, not on some sordid loo seat in a thinly partitioned public lavatory. Some of the best and most natural laxatives are dried fruit, particularly figs and prunes. If you have an existing constipation problem you might like to pack these as part of your hospital kit.

Colic and Crying Babies

This is strictly a past-the-first-week problem, but I am including it as it was often mentioned by our respondents. Colic is a condition in which the baby cries incessantly, drawing up the legs as if in pain. It usually starts after a couple of weeks or so, and the general pattern is that it sets in at its most ferocious – when your baby refuses to be comforted and howls continuously – in the early evening; precisely the time when you are most in need of relaxation. However, some babies are far more badly affected and cry for a good part of the day as well. It's called three-month colic because by three months most babies have grown out of it. There are all sorts of theories about this very common condition, including an immature gut, food intolerance and the rest, although very few of these theories have any science behind them. Because it is a condition of theories, there are no treatments which are soundly based, and in any case when the condition gets better is it because of the treatment, or would it have got better anyway? Sometimes colicky babies are those whose mothers have a huge supply of milk, which just gushes into the baby, meaning that the baby takes in a lot of air too. Regulating your flow by expressing a bit first may help, and if you have a bottle fed baby try a change of teat, perhaps to one with a reduced flow. Anything is worth a try. Anti-spasmodic medicines including gripe water may help but equally may bring no relief. You might try the two homeopathic remedies, fennel and camomile, which can work amazingly well for some babies, although do nothing for others. I did a film with *Tomorrow's World* about the use of cranial osteopathy, a variant of normal osteopathy, for colic. Many parents reported success and you can certainly try this, but I wasn't wholly convinced.

The effect on you of a continuously crying baby can be devastating. Part of it is that you feel completely helpless – your baby seems in evident pain, yet you can do nothing to help. All the soothing and comforting you give are to no avail. So, in addition to exhaustion and feeling a failure as a mother, you may also have quite murderous feelings about harming your offspring, which may alarm you and further diminish your sense of self-worth as a mother. I personally think that such feelings are entirely understandable and natural – the problems start when you really do pick up your baby and shake it, rather than just thinking about it (shaking may not seem like much, but it can cause brain damage in a small baby).

The first thing to say is that an end is in sight – it will pass. The second is that time out sometimes helps: periods of around twenty minutes when you shut the bedroom door on the baby, safe in the cot, and just let it cry whilst you try and concentrate on doing something else for yourself. If you are in a small flat and can't get away, even this can be difficult. I resorted to taking my first baby out in the car or out for a walk because it was the only thing that seemed to quieten him down in the evening.

I don't think you should underestimate just how demoralising it can be to have a baby who cries continuously, from colic or anything else. You need as much help as you can get, and an organisation like Cry-Sis is your first step because they know exactly what you are going through and can suggest a range of ways to counteract crying. You can take your baby to the GP or health visitor if you are worried that the crying might be symptomatic of some underlying problem, but I am afraid that usually it isn't. You just have a baby that cries a great deal. It can seem very unfair and you do need support from outside – not just from your partner, but friends and family who can take the baby for a couple of hours and let you relax, or let off steam.

You need to develop strategies for stopping the crying. These must be changed frequently, because what works one day might not work the next. Try parking the pram (covered with a net to stop cats) underneath a tree or beneath the washing line so that your baby can watch the shapes of leaves and washing moving. Experiment with jiggling the baby about to find out what is soothing – each baby is different. You can tell how automatic this has become with mothers if you go to the supermarket and see a woman jiggling her trolley. I bet you a dollar to a doughnut she has a baby at home. If you have the sort of baby that cries when left alone, invest in a sling and attach the baby whilst you go about your daily routine – and hang the people who tell you that it's 'spoiling' the baby. You're the one whose life is being spoilt. And if sitting your baby in front of the telly produces some quiet, then do it and don't feel guilty.

Going Back to Work

Some women who are completely convinced that they will want to return to work fail to do so having had a baby. Some women can't wait to get back to work. For most, getting back to work is a financial necessity and can involve the most heart-wrenching of decisions. For further details of benefits that you could or should be claiming during this period, you should contact your local Citizens Advice Bureau or Association for Improvement in the Maternity Services. You can always try the local benefits office, but they are not generally as helpful as they might be. What is sure is that benefits and maternity pay are not enough; but women have always been penalised for having babies. I think that this situation, now that more women are having babies in their thirties rather than in their twenties, will change, especially as professional women are becoming an increasingly large proportion of the workforce.

For the present, however, going back to work isn't easy. You may find yourself trying to be all things to all people – efficient at work, on top of the housework and a dutiful mother and wife – and finding, as I did, that you feel you are doing none of them well and are constantly exhausted. I think this feeling is entirely undestandable, and rather than railing against it and making yourself feel worse in the process, or putting even more effort into everything, you should come to terms with your situation. Accept that life is not ideal and go with the flow. Try and involve your partner and get him to realise what a problem it is for you, enlist his help and that of your friends. If you can afford to have someone come and do the housework, even for a couple of hours a week, do it and don't feel guilty – some things just have to give and it might as well be the ironing. And do please try to do something for yourself, be it a bit of exercise, a drink after work, some pointless shopping or whatever, every week. For by doing something for yourself instead of feeling that you are constantly working on others' behalf you will give yourself the tonic and self-respect you so desperately need at this stage.

Fatigue

And then there is the exhaustion. This was a point brought up by nearly two-thirds of mothers in our survey.

> 'I wish I'd known just how tired I was going to be. I would have rested a bit more.'

> 'Get all the sleep you can now, you'll be short of sleep for a long time yet.'

'Why did I think that babies slept at night?'

Almost every respondent in our survey said exactly the same thing. In a nutshell their advice was simple – if this is your first pregnancy, you'll never have it so good again, rest while you can. I remember when I was pregnant the first time. I was so full of energy that I couldn't think of resting. I decorated, did a full-time job and was ready to clean the windows when I got home. Looking back on it, my husband must have been in despair. However active and get-up-and-go you feel in late pregnancy, getting lots of rest is very sound indeed. The process of birth, particularly if you have a caesarean, which is after all a major operation not just a quick snip, takes it out of you. Even if you didn't have a baby to look after you'd still be completely wiped out by the experience.

I have to tell you that exhaustion is pretty much the common ground of parents of children of any age, but it can seem life-sapping in those first couple of weeks after your baby is born. There are all sorts of ways to cope with it. One of the best is just to go with the flow and not try to be superwoman. If the house is looking a tip, don't worry; housework (as many of our correspondents said) will wait. Even if you hate having your mum in the house, do accept her help, or indeed the help and support of anyone who offers it. Try and put off having visitors (it will mean cleaning up or cooking, or just being nice, when all you want to do is crash out). Rest – and this is really important – when the baby is resting, whatever time of day that is. And don't whatever you do wake up your baby to feed her, especially last thing at night in the hope that it will mean your baby will sleep through, because she won't and it will just mean extra effort. Try to eat well – you need it – and don't feel guilty if you live for a couple of weeks on ready-prepared meals from the supermarket. I say all of this because exhaustion is your worst enemy and the one that I think pushes many women over the edge.

If all this seems like a potent brew, you are right. Most mothers feel pretty low in the first couple of months. Is this postnatal depression, or is it just how all mothers feel? It is pretty much the latter, compounded by tiredness and perhaps also exacerbated by some of the changes in lifestyle that have been forced upon you if one of you has given up work and there is one less income. You will find that things gradually get better, that you find coping easier and that you begin to enjoy your baby more of the time instead of seeing her as a constant chore. It will help you enormously to talk to other women in the same position, and frankly just getting out of the house for a while can be bliss in itself. One of the best ways to get through this period is to be a joiner – join postnatal exercise classes, mother and baby groups, mother and baby swimming classes, whatever. Be frank about how you are feeling and you will soon discover that far from being a non-coper, you are actually just the same as (sometimes rather better than, which may give you a lift) other women in the same boat. You will also find that you can recruit a babysitter from the ranks of other new mothers, knowing that they have the skills to cope with your baby. This can be very reassuring and may allow you and your partner some very much needed time to yourselves.

Depression

Birth is such a momentous event in your life that it is almost bound to be followed by a sense of anti-climax. All those soft-focus pictures of slim, pretty, immaculate mothers with soft-focus babies create a very romantic picture of how life with a newborn baby is going to be. There probably are some moments like that, and there are feelings of great tenderness and contentment – a bit like, if I can use a pre-birth analogy, when you've got all the ironing and shopping done, the house looks clean and tidy, the supper is cooking quietly and everything is peaceful; know that feeling? Life with a demanding new baby can seem very different to how you had imagined it. For a start you will find that an extraordinary amount of your time is spent on doing things with and for the baby and there is no time for anything else. Your washing machine will go into overdrive (babies get through impossible amounts of laundry even in a day), your hands will be chapped and sore (from constant handwashing before feeding, after changing, etc.) and once you have completed one set of tasks, for instance feeding and changing, never mind the housework, it seems another round of the same tasks starts again.

The trouble is that it's not like the house clean, ironing done analogy, because you can always live in a mess and wear clothes that don't need ironing, or live on takeaways if you want, thus delaying the inevitable and giving yourself a breather. You simply can't do that with a baby – they have to be fed, have to be changed, have to have their clothes washed or else you would run out in a trice and have to sit them in Jiffy bags. It's the sense of the relentless demand, and being completely tied to this baby, that gets to many women. And one thing that is never really explained is that babies do not smile much for at least six weeks, so all your effort is not rewarded with smiles; tiny babies can't even put their arms around you and hug you.

Another problem about the soft-focus mum bit is that it paints a portrait of motherhood in which you look your best very quickly. Most women look pretty awful for the first three months or so. In addition to leaking from every orifice, that pregnancy glow and sheen has disappeared. Your hair will be, in all likelihood, coming out in handfuls, you may be rather spotty from all those hormone changes and your clothes may feel downright uncomfortable because you still have quite a bit of weight to lose. You may not feel as fit as you did, not just because of exhaustion but because you do not get the same opportunities for fitness regimes that you had before the birth. And some of those pick-me-up standbys, like buying yourself new clothes, are denied to you, partly because you are still in the Mighty Morphin stage when buying a 14 seems pointless when you hope to be a 12 next week, and partly because you have now discovered that shopping with a baby is one of the most gruesome tasks known.

You may have quite different feelings than you had expected, too. You may have slipped very easily into the role of motherhood, or you may be feeling confused and overwhelmed, wondering what has hit you and seriously questioning why you, a sensible grown-up woman, could ever have thought that parenthood seemed like a good lifeplan. You may be feeling very isolated, especially in the early hours of the morning as your baby wakes yet again, and wondering how much more of this you can cope with. Your relationship with your partner may be very close, yet you may wonder, as he escapes to work every day, why he doesn't seem to understand exactly what you are going through, how much time it all takes and why you feel so down, when he is still pretty elated by it all.

In addition, you may meet other mothers and instead of feeling supported, feel guilty because they seem to be coping so well, when you are still in your dressing gown at lunchtime and have a baby that cries all the time. And sometimes, and this is almost hardest to bear, when you most want someone to cosset that battered, leaking body of yours, take you out, be nice to you, tell you how wonderful you look, fancy you even – all they want to do is coo over the baby, completely ignoring you.

But where does mild depression, very common and understandable in women following childbirth, stop and a more serious form of postnatal depression start? About 80 per cent of women will have the so-called baby blues, usually starting at about the third or fourth day after the birth. Uncontrolled weeping, being quite irrational and having wild mood swings are the symptoms, but these rapidly resolve, if not within a couple of days, then usually within ten days. For about 1 in 10 women, the feelings of not being able to cope are overwhelming and do not get better. Although they may be very good at caring for their babies, they tend to avoid eye contact and do not play much with them. They tend to wake very early, have very strong feelings of being completely worthless and inadequate and may find completing even the simplest of tasks a trial. There may be outbursts of irrational anger or weeping, acute anxiety or obsessions about the baby's health or welfare. They may become more and more house-bound, fearing going out and not wanting to meet other mums, because they feel that this will only reinforce their feelings of low esteem. They may either overeat or undereat. One of the features of postnatal depression that has struck me has been the way in which sufferers manage to persuade almost everyone around them, bar perhaps their partner or closest friends, that they are fine and coping well. Sometimes this just further delays treatment. There isn't a set time at which postnatal depression sets in, although you should be alert to the possibility for up to a year. You may find, particularly if your baby had a very dramatic start to life, perhaps requiring months of special care, that you cope well until the baby comes home and only then does the full enormity of what you have been through sink in, and depression hit you. If any of these feelings are ones you recognise either in yourself or in your partner, then help is urgently needed.

At one level, you can contact some of the support groups, such as the Postnatal Illness Association (see Appendix I), but you may need more sustained support in the form of therapy. Some GPs can direct you to NHS counselling, although not all areas have such facilities. The British Association of Counsellors can recommend someone in your area who is qualified to help, although you will have to pay for this, and it may be that a bit of one-to-one reassurance is all that you require. On the other hand, it may be more helpful for you to see your GP and to have drug therapy. You may feel slightly horrified by this, because you feel (and you might be alone in this) that you don't have a problem severe enough to warrant medication, and because you fear being on drugs for a very long time. Although drugs do take a while to work, they can be immensely helpful, allowing you a breathing space from the severest of your symptoms.

You don't have to be a particular 'type' of person to have postnatal depression, nor do you have to have a history of mental illness or depression. In fact, it is often copers who seem to be hit worst. Some circumstances will make postnatal depression more likely: a very difficult delivery which you have not found it easy to come to terms with; very little support; difficult circumstances during pregnancy and in the post-birth period with relationships, house moves, bereavement of a parent. However, many women in appallingly difficult circumstances do not develop postnatal depression. There are certainly two schools of thought about the cause of PND – one is that it is caused by the sort of lifestyle changes that I have outlined, the other that PND is hormonal in origin. There is probably an element of both. The important thing is not to let PND get out of hand, as the sooner treatment of whatever form is instituted, the easier it is to deal with.

There is a third sort of postnatal illness – puerperal psychosis. It affects about 1 in 1,000 mothers, involves mania, delusions and suicidal feelings, and is terrifying – and frighteningly obvious – to everyone in contact with the mother. Immediate hospitalisation and drug treatment is essential, preferably at one of the specialist mother and baby units which are sadly so sparsely provided in the UK. The good news is that most mothers will make a complete recovery. If you have had PND before, you are more likely to get it in a subsequent pregnancy, but this is certainly not a foregone conclusion, and is something that you need to discuss with your GP in advance of your next pregnancy.

In some ways, concluding this book with an extreme of postnatal life is unfortunate, because despite the exhaustion, despite not looking or feeling your best, despite not being quite sure sometimes that you haven't made a terrible mistake, you can still be quite overwhelmed when you look at that baby of yours. If you find yourself crying tears of joy as you stand over her cot, thinking just how special she is and how very lucky you are to have her, you will be doing what hundreds of thousands of other mothers are doing, or will be doing, as their babies grow up. And just one moment like this can make up for everything else. Enjoy it.

Appendix I

Useful Addresses

Place of Birth

Association for Improvements in the Maternity Services (AIMS)
40 Kingswood Avenue
London NW6 6LS
tel. 0181 960 5585

Support and advice about parents' rights and choices within maternity services, including home births.

Independent Midwives Association
Nightingale Cottage
Shamblehurst Lane
Botley
Hants SO3 2BY
tel. 01703 694429

Advice about home birth. Can put you in touch with local independent midwife.

Society to Support Home Confinements
Lydgate
Wolsingham
Co Durham DL13 3HA
tel. 01388 528044

Maternity Benefits

Maternity Alliance
15 Britannia Street
London WC1X 9JP
tel. 0171 837 1265

Association of Breast Feeding Mothers
26 Hornsham Close
London SE26 4PH
tel. 0181 778 4769

La Leche League
PO Box BM3424
London WC1N 3XX
tel. 0171 242 1278

Also **National Childbirth Trust** (see under Specialist
Support Organisations)

Specialist Support Organisations

Action on Pre-Eclampsia (APEC)
31–33 College Road
Harrow
Middx
tel. 01923 266778

Aqua Birth Pools
Active Birth Centre
55 Dartmouth Road Park
London NW5 1SL
tel. 0171 267 3006

For hire of birthing pools and also information about active birth.

Association for Postnatal Illness
25 Jerdan Place
London SW6 1BE
tel. 0171 386 0868

Particularly effective support group, with advice given by women who have themselves suffered from postnatal depression.

Association for Spina Bifida and Hydrocephalus (ASBAH)
42 Park House
Peterborough PE1 2UQ
tel. 01753 555988

BLISS
17–21 Emerald Street
London WC1N 3QL
tel. 0171 831 9393

Support and information for parents with babies in special care.

British Association of Counsellors
1 Regent Place
Rugby
War
tel. 01788 578328

British Diabetic Association
10 Queen Anne Street
London W1M 0BD
tel. 0171 323 1531

Support if you are diabetic and either pregnant or wanting to
conceive.

British Homeopathic Association
27a Devonshire Street
London W1N 4RJ
tel. 0171 935 2163

Advice for homeopathy.
(Also Faculty of Homeopathy, 0171 837 9469, has register of
homeopaths.)

Caesarean Support Network
2 Hurst Park Drive
Huyton
Liverpool L36 1TF
tel. 01151 480 1184

Cervical Stitch Network
Fairfield
Wolverton Road
North Lindsey
War CV35 8LA
tel. 0192684 3223

Information about cervical stitch used to prevent late miscarriage.

Child Bereavement Trust
1 Millside
Riversdale
Bourne End
Bucks SL8 5EB

For written advice only. Provides support, resources and information for bereaved families who lose children at any stage of their lives.

CHILD
PO Box 154
Hounslow
Middx TW5 0EZ
tel. 0181 893 7110

Advice on problems conceiving.

CONTACT A FAMILY
70 Tottenham Court Road
London W1P 0HA
tel. 0171 383 3555

Outstandingly helpful organisation who can direct you to advice and support on specific conditions in children, such as heart disease as well as rare syndromes.

Council for Complementary Medicine
179 Gloucester Place
London NW1 6DX
tel. 0171 724 9103

Information on all forms of alternative medicine.

Cry-Sis
BM Cry-Sis
London WC1N 3XX
tel. 0171 404 5011

Help for parents whose babies cry excessively.

Cystic Fibrosis Research Trust
Alexandra House
5 Blyth Road
Bromley BR1 3RS
tel. 0181 464 7211

For information about cystic fibrosis and about carrier testing.

Down's Syndrome Association
155 Mitcham Road
London SW17 9PG
tel. 0181 682 4001

Down's Syndrome Screening Service
St James's University Hospital
Leeds LS9 7TF
tel. 01532 344013

Eating in pregnancy helpline:
tel. 0114 242 4084

Advice on nutrition before, during and after pregnancy from experts.

Family Planning Association
27–35 Mortimer Street
London W1N 7RJ
tel. 0171 636 7866

Particularly good on contraceptive choices after birth.

Foresight
28 The Paddock
Godalming
Surrey GU7 1XD
tel. 01483 427839

Pre-conceptual organisation.

Foundation for the Study of Infant Deaths
14 Halkin Street
London SW1X 7DD
tel. 0171 235 0965

Cot death advice and reassurance.

Genetic Interest Group
25–29 Farringdon Road
London EC1M 3JB
tel. 01865 744002

Will give you information on regional genetic centres (for genetic testing and advice).

Meet a Mum (MAMA)

58 Malden Avenue
South Norwood
London SE25 4HS
tel. 0181 656 7318

Help for all new mothers, especially those with postnatal depression.

Miscarriage Association

c/o Clayton Hospital
Northgate
Wakefield
W. Yorks WF1 3JS
tel. 01924 200799

Multiple Births Foundation

Queen Charlotte's Hospital
Goldhawk Road
London W6 0XG
tel. 0181 740 3519

Advice and support for mothers of twins and more.

National Association of Medical Herbalists

56 Longbrook Street
Exeter EX4 6AH
tel. 01392 426022

Can provide list of members. Do not attempt DIY herbalism during pregnancy — seek proper advice.

National Childbirth Trust
Alexander House
Oldham Terrace
Acton
London W3 6NH
tel. 0181 992 8637

Advice and literature on antenatal classes, breast feeding and much more.

QUIT
Victory House
170 Tottenham Court Road
London W1P 0HA
tel. 0171 487 3000

Practical advice for would-be non-smokers.

Royal College of Obstetricians and Gynaecologists
27 Sussex Place
Regent's Park
London NW1 4RG
tel. 0171 262 5425

Support around Termination for Abnormality (SATFA)
73–75 Charlotte Street
London W1P 1LB
tel. 0171 631 0280

Will offer advice on antenatal testing, as well as support for those facing termination for abnormality. Excellent source of information and help.

Stillbirth and Neonatal Death Association (SANDS)
28 Portland Place
London W1N 4DE
tel. 0171 436 7940

Support and information network for parents faced with the loss of a baby.

Toxoplasmosis Trust
61–71 Collier Street
London N1 9BE
tel. 0171 713 0599

WellBeing
27 Sussex Place
Regent's Park
London NW1 4SP
tel. 0171 262 5337
Helpline: 0891 518911
(Sun 10–4 only)

Organisation funding research into women's health, including pregnancy, birth, prematurity and infertility.

Women's Health and Reproductive Rights
52–54 Featherstone Street
London EC1Y 8RT
tel. 0171 251 6333 (working hours, not Tues)

Best source of information on women's health, bar none.

Colgate Medical Services
Shirley Avenue
Windsor
SR4 5LH
tel. 01753 860378

Supply sets of 3 weighted cones (Femina 3) for pelvic toning.
About £25 by mail order.

Appendix II

Further Reading

Robert Winston, *Getting Pregnant*, Pan, 1993.

Iain Chalmers et al., *Effective Care in Pregnancy and Childbirth*, Oxford University Press, 1990.

Fiona Ford, Robert Fraser and Hilary Dimond, *Healthy Eating for You and Your Baby*, Pan, 1994.

I. Kohn and P.-L. Moffit, *A Silent Sorrow: Pregnancy Loss*, Headway, 1994.
M. Leroy, *Miscarriage*, Macdonald Optima, 1988.
C. Moulder, *Miscarriage, Women's Experiences and Needs*, Pandora, 1992.
A. Oakley, A. McPherson and H. Roberts, *Miscarriage*, Penguin, 1990.

Ros Kane, *The Cervical Stitch: What it is Like* (via the Miscarriage Association).

Chris Redman and Isabel Walker, *Pre-Eclampsia: The Facts*, Oxford University Press, 1992.

Melissa Brooks, *Caesarean Birth*, Optima, 1989.
Dr. C. Francome, Prof. W. Savage et al., *Caesarean Birth in Britain*, Middlesex University Press, 1993 (and via the NCT).

Appendix III

Practical Parenting Survey: The Results

This questionnaire, headed 'What Worries Mums to Be?', appeared in *Practical Parenting* magazine in March 1994. Nearly 10,000 women replied. The key findings were surprising:

42% felt they were not prepared for what happened during birth.

60% of mothers-to-be find pregnancy a worrying time; 80% were 'anxious'.

35% found that the attitudes of health professionals made it difficult for them to share their worries.

80% would prefer to know what can go wrong during pregnancy and birth.

60% got all or most of their information about pregnancy from books.

Here are the questions with the breakdown of the findings:

IF YOU ARE PREGNANT NOW, WAS THIS PREGNANCY . . .?

% based on those who are pregnant now (339 respondents)

Planned	75
Accidental	19
Aided	2

Three quarters of those who were pregnant at the time of completing their questionnaire reported that this pregnancy was planned. Almost one fifth described their current pregnancy as accidental, while only a very small proportion reported that this pregnancy was aided.

Only a little over two thirds of those aged under 25 reported that this pregnancy was planned.

Married respondents were substantially more likely to report that their pregnancy was planned. A little over four fifths of married respondents reported that this pregnancy was planned, compared to just less than three fifths of those living with their partner, and slightly more than two fifths of single respondents.

Single respondents were most likely to report that this pregnancy was accidental. Well over half of these reported that their pregnancy was accidental.

IF YOU ARE PREGNANT NOW, HOW LONG DID IT TAKE YOU TO GET PREGNANT?

% based on those who are pregnant now (339 respondents)

Less than 6 months	73
Up to 1 year	13
More than 1 year but less than 2 years	4
2 years or more	6

Almost three quarters of those who were pregnant at the time of completing their questionnaire reported that it had taken less than six months to get pregnant. Just over one tenth reported that it had taken up to one year to get pregnant, while for one tenth it had taken more than one year.

IF YOU ARE PREGNANT NOW, WHERE ARE YOU PLANNING TO GIVE BIRTH?

% based on those who are pregnant now (339 respondents)

At home	3
In a GP unit in hospital	6
In a hospital maternity unit	89

The overwhelming majority of those who were pregnant at the time of completing their questionnaire were planning to give birth in a hospital maternity unit

Regionally, those living in the Midlands and East Anglia were slightly more likely to be planning to give birth at home or in a GP unit in hospital.

HAVE ANY OF YOUR PREVIOUS PREGNANCIES ENDED IN MISCARRIAGE OR THE LOSS OF THE BABY?

	%
Yes	26
No	72

About one quarter of sample members reported that one or more of their previous pregnancies had ended in miscarriage or the loss of the baby. It is not, however, possible to determine the proportion of respondents for which this question is not applicable.

Those who reported that they found pregnancy a worrying time were more likely than other respondents to have experienced miscarriage or the loss of a baby.

IF YES, HOW MANY?

% based on those who have previously miscarried or lost a
baby (266 respondents)

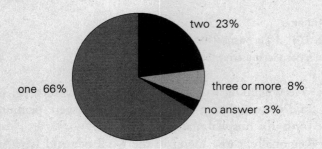

Approximately two thirds of those who had experienced
miscarriage, or lost a baby, reported that this had occurred
once. Almost one quarter of these respondents reported that
they had experienced miscarriage, or loss of a baby, in two
pregnancies, while less than one tenth had experienced such
events in three or more pregnancies.

On average, these respondents had experienced either
miscarriage or loss of a baby in 1.41 pregnancies.

WOULD YOU SAY THAT IN GENERAL YOU ARE . . .?

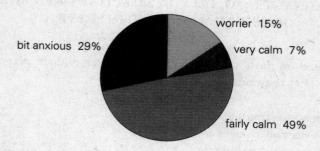

worrier 15%

very calm 7%

bit anxious 29%

fairly calm 49%

While less than one tenth of this sample described themselves as 'very calm', almost half described themselves as 'fairly calm'. Over one quarter of respondents considered that they were generally 'a bit anxious', and almost one sixth described themselves as 'a worrier'.

Those who found pregnancy a worrying time were substantially more likely than other respondents to describe themselves as either 'a bit anxious' or 'a worrier'.

ARE YOU FINDING, OR DID YOU FIND, PREGNANCY A WORRYING TIME?

	%
Yes	57
No	42

Well over half of respondents were finding, or had found, pregnancy a worrying time. Over four fifths of those who described themselves as 'a worrier' were finding, or had found, pregnancy a worrying time.

IF YOU ALREADY HAVE CHILDREN AND ARE PREGNANT NOW, DO YOU SEEM TO WORRY MORE OR LESS THAN YOU DID IN PREVIOUS PREGNANCIES?

% based on those who already have children and are pregnant now (194 respondents)

I'm worrying more this time	34
I'm worrying the same amount	29
I'm worrying less this time	35

Respondents were divided fairly evenly in terms of how much they were worrying this time compared to previous pregnancies. Slightly more than one third of those with children who were pregnant at the time of completing this questionnaire were worrying less this time, while almost the same proportion were worrying more this time. Those aged over 30 were slightly more likely to report that they were worrying more this time.

IS THERE ANYTHING YOU ARE ENJOYING/DID ENJOY ABOUT BEING PREGNANT?

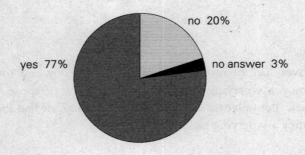

More than three quarters of sample members were enjoying, or had enjoyed, something about being pregnant.

IF YES, WHAT?

% based on those answering yes (774 respondents)

Feeling the baby move/kick	30
The attention received	12
Feeling well/healthy	11
The idea that I'm creating a new life	10
Everything/all of it	9
Feeling special/important	8
Feeling/watching the baby grow	7
My shape/getting fat	5
Being pampered/spoilt	4
The excitement	4
The anticipation	4
Being able to eat whatever I like	4
Feeling happy/content	3
People's interest/concern	3
Seeing baby on scan/hearing the heartbeat	3
Making plans/preparations	3

Nearly one third of these respondents answered that they were enjoying, or had enjoyed, feeling the baby move and kick. In the region of one tenth were enjoying, or had enjoyed, the attention received, feeling well/feeling healthy, and the idea that they were creating a new life.

DID YOU FIND YOURSELF DOING ANYTHING TOTALLY OUT OF CHARACTER WHILE YOU WERE PREGNANT?

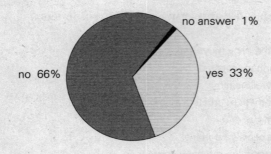

no answer 1%

no 66%

yes 33%

One third of sample members had found themselves doing something totally out of character while they were pregnant.

IF YES, WHAT?

% based on those answering yes (329 respondents)

Being forgetful/poor memory	29
Emotional/crying	21
Food cravings/eating weird things	9
Doing housework/cleaning constantly	8
Short/bad tempered	7
Doing/saying silly things	6
Sleeping a lot/day time naps	4
Mood swings	4
Ate constantly/big appetite	3
Clumsy/dropping things	3
Full of life/lots of energy	2
Slowed down/less energy	2

Unable to concentrate/think	2
Aggressive/violent behaviour	2
Unable to sleep	2

Well over one quarter of these respondents reported that they were forgetful or suffered from a poor memory while pregnant. A little over one fifth reported that they felt emotional or tended to cry more frequently while pregnant.

DID YOU HAVE ANY STRANGE FOOD CRAVINGS WHILE PREGNANT?

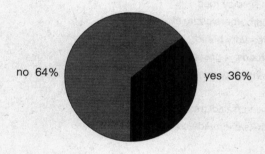

no 64%   yes 36%

Just over one third of sample members had strange food cravings while pregnant.

IF YES, WHAT?

% based on those answering yes (363 respondents)

Fruit/oranges/lemons/bananas, etc.	17
Pickles/pickled onions/pickled gherkins, etc.	12
Ice cream/ice lollies	9

Chocolate/chocolate bars	7
Sweets/jelly babies/sherbet dips, etc.	6
Crisps	6
Fish/shellfish	6
Other vegetables/carrots/raw vegetables	6
Milk/milkshakes	5
Ice/ice cubes	5
Potato/mash/chips	5
Cheese/cottage cheese	5
Unusual combination sandwiches	5
Fruit juice/orange juice/tomato juice, etc.	4
Salad/tomato/cucumber/lettuce, etc.	4
Curry/chilli/spicy food	4
Fast food/burgers/pizza, etc.	4
Toast/bread/dry bread	4
All non foods, e.g. soap/coal, etc.	4
Vinegar/vinegary things	3
Biscuits	3
Mayonnaise/salad cream	3
Fizzy drinks/cherryade/cola, etc.	3

About one sixth of these respondents craved fruit, particularly oranges, lemons or bananas, and slightly more than one tenth craved pickles or pickled foods, particularly onions or gherkins.

WHAT, IF ANYTHING, WORRIED YOU DURING PREGNANCY?

	Mean score	% very worried	Did it happen? (% yes)
Health of baby	3.78	36	5
Miscarriage	3.26	28	12
Food, drink, medicines taken in pregnancy	2.73	12	8
Bleeding	2.62	16	23
Putting on weight you wouldn't lose	2.57	13	20
Having to be induced	2.30	10	20
Antenatal tests	2.19	8	9
Going into labour early	2.10	8	11
High blood pressure	2.00	6	16

Respondents worried most during pregnancy about the health of their baby. Over one third were 'very worried' about the health of their baby, and this achieved the highest mean score, where a score of 5 represents 'very worried' and a score of 1 represents 'not worried'. Over one quarter of respondents were 'very worried' about miscarriage, and one sixth were 'very worried' about bleeding during pregnancy.

Almost one quarter of respondents had experienced bleeding during pregnancy, one fifth had been induced, and the same proportion considered that they had put on weight that they wouldn't lose. One sixth of this sample had experienced high blood pressure during pregnancy.

ANY OTHER WORRY?

Other worries during pregnancy reported by small proportions of respondents included: the prospect of having to have a caesarean, worries about stillbirth, fear of labour/giving birth and the pain involved, including tearing, episiotomy, and having to have stitches, lack of baby movements, worries about going into hospital, and general worries about how they would cope with the newborn baby.

WHAT, IF ANYTHING, WORRIED YOU ABOUT THE BIRTH?

	Mean score	% very worried	Did it happen? (% yes)
Whether you'd cope during labour	3.18	24	14
Needing an assisted delivery	2.91	15	14
Having a caesarean	2.80	20	11
Birth not going as planned	2.77	15	20
Pain relief in labour	2.66	13	17
Not being able to hold your baby immediately	2.40	10	13
Whether your partner would cope	2.16	7	8
Not having a familiar midwife/doctor	1.85	5	15
Place of birth	1.56	4	3

Respondents worried most about whether they would cope during labour. Almost one quarter were 'very worried' about this. Worries about coping during labour achieved the highest mean score, where a score of 5 represents 'very worried' and a score of 1 represents 'not worried'. One fifth of respondents were 'very worried' about having a caesarean, and nearly one sixth were 'very worried' about needing an assisted delivery, and the birth not going as planned.

One fifth of respondents reported that the birth of a child had not gone as planned.

ANY OTHER WORRY?

Other worries about the birth reported by small proportions of respondents included: worries about stillbirth or the baby dying, fear of bowel movements in labour, and worries about not getting to hospital in time.

IF YOU ALREADY HAVE A BABY, DO YOU FEEL THAT YOU WERE PREPARED FOR WHAT HAPPENED DURING THE BIRTH?

% based on those who already have children (865 respondents)

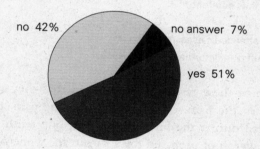

no 42%   no answer 7%

yes 51%

A little over half of those with children already felt that they were prepared for what happened during the birth. Just over two fifths felt that they were not prepared for what happened.

Generally, as one might have expected, those with more children were more likely to report that they felt they were prepared. Well over half of those with two children, and two thirds of those with three or more children felt that they were prepared for what happened during the birth.

IF NO, WHY NOT?

% based on those who do not feel that they were prepared for what happened during the birth (367 respondents)

The pain/intensity of pain	16
Caesarean/emergency caesarean	14
Nothing can prepare you/cannot be prepared for the unknown	10
Very quick/short labour	7
Very slow/long labour	7
Premature baby/born very early	4
Baby in distress/complications	4
Every birth is different	4
Induced	4
Had not attended classes/enough classes	3
Poor/insufficient information from classes	3

One sixth of these respondents reported that they were not prepared for the pain, or the intensity of the pain, that they experienced during the birth. More than one tenth reported that they were not prepared for a caesarean, while one tenth suggested that nothing can prepare you for the birth experience.

DID YOU SHARE WORRIES WITH ANYONE?

	%
Yes	80
No	14

The vast majority of respondents, four fifths, shared their worries with someone. Married respondents, and those who were living with their partner but not married, were substantially more likely than single respondents to have shared their worries.

IF YES, WHO WITH?

% based on those who shared their worries (812 respondents)

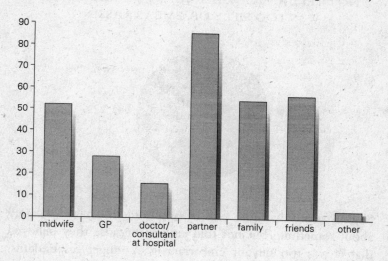

The overwhelming majority of these respondents (87%) shared their worries with their partner. Nine tenths of married respondents, and about the same proportion of those living with their partner but not married, shared their worries with their partner. Interestingly, those with more children were less likely to share their worries with their partner. Only just over three quarters of respondents with three or more children shared their worries with their partner, compared to a little more than nine tenths of those expecting their first child.

Well over half of these respondents shared their worries with friends (56%), family (55%), or with a midwife (53%).

Only just one quarter of these respondents shared their worries with their GP (27%), and just less than one sixth (15%) shared them with a doctor or consultant at the hospital.

DID YOU EVER WORRY ABOUT SOMETHING BUT NOT TELL ANYONE BECAUSE YOU THOUGHT IT WAS TOO SILLY OR EMBARRASSING?

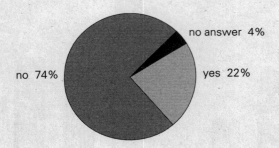

no answer 4%

no 74%

yes 22%

Slightly more than one fifth of sample members had worried about something but not told anyone because they believed that it was too silly or embarrassing. Younger respondents, particularly those aged under 25, were most likely not to have told anyone for this reason.

Almost one third of those who described themselves as 'a worrier' had worried about something but not told anyone, compared to only a little over one tenth of those who considered themselves to be 'very calm'.

IF YES, WHAT WAS IT?

% based on those who worried about something but didn't tell anyone (226 respondents)

Bowel movement in labour	17
Health of baby/deformity/disability	13
Labour/the birth	5
Wetting myself/incontinence	4
Discharge	3
Piles	3
Breast feeding	3
Still birth	3
Bleeding	3
Not being able to cope with baby	3

About one sixth of these respondents worried about opening their bowels during labour, and more than one tenth worried about the health of their baby but did not tell anyone because they believed that it was too silly.

Other answers, provided by small proportions of respondents, included: whether they would love the baby, fear of the baby dying/cot death, lack of baby movement, worries about having to have an episiotomy, and worries about having examinations/internals.

WOULD YOU PREFER NOT TO KNOW WHAT COULD GO WRONG DURING PREGNANCY?

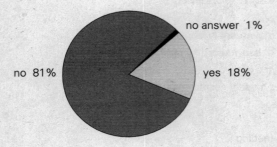

Only a little less than one fifth of sample members reported that they would prefer not to know what could go wrong during pregnancy. The overwhelming majority, just over four fifths of respondents, said that they would prefer to know what could go wrong.

Those who described themselves as 'a bit anxious' or 'a worrier' were slightly more likely to report that they would prefer not to know what could go wrong than those who considered themselves generally to be 'very calm' or 'fairly calm'.

DID YOU EXPERIENCE ANY OF THE FOLLOWING FEARS DURING PREGNANCY?

	Mean score	% very worried	Did it happen? (% yes)
Financial problems	2.84	15	18
Coping as a parent	2.59	15	11
Partner's feelings about you changing	2.28	8	6
Effects on your sex life	2.27	7	22
Loss of freedom	2.13	6	21
Bonding with your baby	2.01	7	9
Career would suffer	1.61	4	9

Respondents worried most about financial problems and coping as a parent. Almost one sixth were 'very worried' about these elements. Worries about financial problems achieved the highest mean score, where a score of 5 represents 'very worried' and a score of 1 represents 'not worried'.

Slightly more than one fifth of respondents reported that their sex life had been affected, and roughly the same proportion had experienced loss of freedom.

ANYTHING ELSE?

Other fears experienced during pregnancy, reported by very small proportions of respondents, included: fears about the health of the baby, sibling jealousy and the reaction of their other children to the new baby, and their partner's reaction to the baby.

HOW WAS YOUR RELATIONSHIP WITH YOUR PARTNER DURING PREGNANCY?

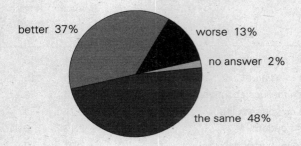

better 37%   worse 13%

no answer 2%

the same 48%

Nearly half of sample members considered that their relationship with their partner is, or was, the same during pregnancy. Half of respondents believed that their relationship with their partner is, or was, different during pregnancy. Almost three quarters of those who reported a difference considered their relationship to be better during pregnancy. A little more than one quarter of those who reported a difference considered their relationship to be worse during pregnancy.

The youngest respondents in this sample were most likely to report that their relationship with their partner was worse during pregnancy.

HOW WAS YOUR SEX LIFE DURING PREGNANCY?

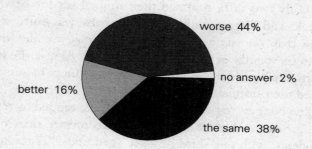

worse 44%

no answer 2%

better 16%

the same 38%

Almost two fifths of sample members considered that their sex life is, or was, the same during pregnancy. Three fifths of respondents believed that their sex life is, or was, different during pregnancy. Almost three quarters of those who reported a difference, considered their sex life to be worse during pregnancy. A little more than one quarter of those who reported a difference considered their sex life to be better during pregnancy.

HOW SOON AFTER YOUR BABY WAS BORN DID YOU RESUME YOUR NORMAL SEX LIFE?

% based on those who have children already (865 respondents)

Less than 6 weeks	27
6 weeks to 3 months	44
3 months to 6 months	14
6 months to 1 year	8
Over 1 year	5

Slightly more than one quarter of those with children resumed their normal sex life less than six weeks after their baby was born. Only two fifths resumed their normal sex life between six weeks and three months after their baby was born, while just less than one sixth resumed their normal sex life within three to six months of the birth of their baby. Almost the same proportion reported that it was six months or more before they resumed their normal sex life.

The youngest respondents in this sample tended to report that they resumed their normal sex life sooner than older respondents, with one third of those aged under 25 resuming their normal sex life within six weeks.

IS YOUR SEX LIFE . . .?

% based on those who have children already (865 respondents)

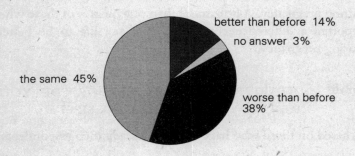

better than before 14%

no answer 3%

the same 45%

worse than before 38%

Approaching half of those with children considered that their sex life is the same now compared to before the birth of their child/children. Just over half of these respondents believed that their sex life has changed. Almost three quarters of those who reported a difference considered their sex life to be worse than it was before the birth. A little more than one quarter of those who reported a difference considered their sex life to be better than it was before the birth.

WHO GAVE YOU, OR IS GIVING YOU, MOST EMOTIONAL SUPPORT DURING PREGNANCY?

	Mean score	% stating most support
Your partner	4.10	52
Your mother	3.67	21
A friend	3.04	9
Midwife or health visitor	3.02	10
GP	2.46	5
Obstetrician	1.77	2

Just over half of this sample considered that their partner is giving, or gave them, the most emotional support during pregnancy. Partner achieved the highest mean score (4.10), where a score of 5 represents most support, and a score of 1 represents least support. Well over half of married respondents, and almost half of those living with their partner but not married, considered that their partner is giving, or gave them, the most emotional support during pregnancy.

A little more than one fifth of respondents considered that their mother is giving, or gave them, the most emotional support during pregnancy. The youngest respondents, particularly those aged under 25, were most likely to endorse 'mother', a little more than one quarter of respondents in this age group considered that their mother is giving, or gave them, the most emotional support (mean score = 3.90).

OTHER?

Others named as 'most supportive', mentioned by small proportions of respondents, included: sister (4%), mother-in-law (1%), father (1%), and other female relatives (aunt, grandmother, sister-in-law, etc.).

WERE YOU HAPPY WITH THE INFORMATION AND ADVICE GIVEN TO YOU BY THE HEALTH PROFESSIONALS WHO LOOKED AFTER YOU DURING PREGNANCY?

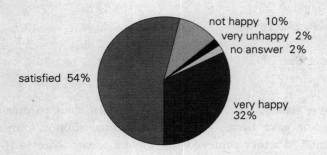

The vast majority of sample members, well over four fifths, were satisfied or very happy with the information and advice given by health professionals looking after them. Almost one third were very happy with the information and advice given to them. A mean score of 1.82 was achieved, where a score of 1 represents 'very happy' and a score of 4 represents 'very unhappy'.

One tenth of respondents were not happy, and only a relatively small proportion were very unhappy with the information and advice given by health professionals looking after them during pregnancy.

DID THE ATTITUDE OF THE HEALTHCARE PROFESSIONALS EVER MAKE IT DIFFICULT FOR YOU TO SHARE YOUR WORRIES WITH THEM?

	%
Yes	35
No	64

A little more than one third of respondents believed that the attitude of healthcare professionals made it difficult to share worries with them.

Over two fifths of those who found pregnancy a worrying time believed that the attitude of healthcare professionals made it difficult to share worries with them.

WHERE DID YOU GET MOST OF YOUR INFORMATION ABOUT PREGNANCY AND BIRTH?

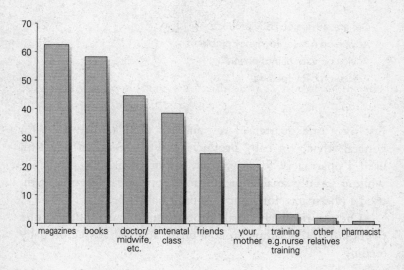

Nearly two thirds of sample members (64%) obtained most of their information about pregnancy from magazines, and almost three fifths (58%) got most of their information from books.

Approaching half of respondents (45%) obtained most of their information from a doctor, midwife, or other medical person, and a little less than two fifths (38%) reported that they got most of their information about pregnancy from antenatal classes.

Almost one quarter of respondents (24%) got most of their information from friends, and slightly more than one fifth (21%) reported that they got most of their information from their mother.

Only a very small proportion (1%) obtained most of their information about pregnancy from a pharmacist.

DID YOU USE A PHARMACIST FOR ANY OF THE FOLLOWING?

	%
General advice on baby products	27
Advice on minor pregnancy problems	19
Advice on your baby's health	17
Advice on baby feeding	5
No answer	51

Just over one quarter of respondents used a pharmacist for general advice on baby products. A little less than one fifth used a pharmacist for advice on minor pregnancy problems, while a slightly smaller proportion, approximately one sixth, used a pharmacist for advice on their baby's health.

Only a relatively small proportion of respondents, one twentieth of this sample, used a pharmacist for advice on baby feeding.

Just over half of sample members did not provide an answer, suggesting that they did not use a pharmacist for any of the above.

HOW OFTEN DID YOU/DO YOU SEEK THE ADVICE OF YOUR PHARMACIST?

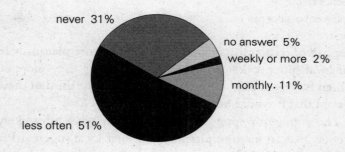

never 31%

no answer 5%

weekly or more 2%

monthly. 11%

less often 51%

Only a very small proportion of respondents sought the advice of their pharmacist weekly or more often. Just over one tenth sought the advice of their pharmacist monthly, while a little more than half reported that they sought his or her advice less often than this.

Nearly one third of this sample never sought the advice of their pharmacist.

IF THERE WAS A PHARMACY IN YOUR LOCAL SUPERMARKET, HOW WOULD THIS INFLUENCE WHERE YOU DO YOUR MAIN SHOPPING FOR YOUR BABY?

	%
Big influence	17
Some influence	37
Little or no influence	44

Over half of respondents reported that an in-store pharmacy in their local supermarket would influence where they shopped for their baby, although only a little less than one third of these believed that it would be a big influence.

The youngest respondents in this sample were most likely to report that an in-store pharmacy in their local supermarket would have a big influence on where they shopped for their baby. Slightly more than one fifth of those aged under 25 believed that it would have a big influence.

More than two fifths of sample members believed that an in-store pharmacy in their local supermarket would have little or no influence on where they did the main shopping for their baby.

IF YOU ALREADY HAVE A BABY, WHAT ONE PIECE OF ADVICE WOULD YOU GIVE TO A WOMAN WHO HAS JUST BECOME PREGNANT?

% based on those who already have children (865 respondents)

Enjoy it/enjoy it while it lasts	27
Get lots of rest/sleep/make the most of the rest	16
Relax/try to relax/learn to relax	10

Don't worry/try not to worry	9
Follow your instincts/listen to your body	6
Find out all you can/get informed	5
Eat sensibly/don't eat too much	4
Take things easy/slow down	4
Ask questions/don't be afraid to ask questions	4
Don't listen to other people's birth horror stories	4
Don't always listen to other people	4
Take one day at a time/each day as it comes	4
Keep an open mind/expect anything	4

Over one quarter of those with children already would advise someone who had just become pregnant to enjoy pregnancy, with most of these recommending that they should 'enjoy it while it lasts'.

One sixth of these respondents would advise someone who had just become pregnant to get plenty of rest and sleep, and to make the most of the opportunity to have plenty of rest before the baby arrives.

One tenth of those with children already stressed the importance of relaxation, recommending that one should learn to relax during pregnancy.

IS THERE ANYTHING YOU WISH YOU'D KNOWN BEFORE YOU GOT PREGNANT?

	%
How tired I would get/about all the sleepless nights	8
How life would change/how much life would be affected	4
What a wonderful experience it is/how good it is	3
How sick I would be/how awful I would feel	3
About the emotional strain/how emotional you feel	3
More about weight control/how hard it is to lose it after	3

How painful/awful labour is	2
About the discomfort/how uncomfortable it is	2
How much hard work is involved	2
How much time is needed/how demanding it is	2
No answer	45

A vast array of both positive and negative responses were offered here. Nearly one tenth of respondents wished that they had known in advance about all the sleepless nights they would experience, and generally how tired they would be throughout.

Well over half of respondents replied that there was something/were things that they wished they had known before becoming pregnant. Just less than half of respondents did not provide an answer here, suggesting that there was nothing in particular that these respondents wished that they had known in advance.

Index